# Basic Anatomy and Physiology in Speech and Hearing

# Basic Anatomy and Physiology in Speech and Hearing

**Carl R. Schneiderman, PhD**
**Department of Speech**
**Communication Disorders Program**
**Washington State University**
**Pullman, Washington**

**College-Hill Press**
**San Diego, California**

**Croom Helm**
**London & Canberra**

College-Hill Press, Inc.
4248 41st Street
San Diego, California 92105

**Library of Congress Cataloging in Publication Data**

Schneiderman, Carl R.
  Basic anatomy and physiology in speech and hearing.

  Bibliography: p
  Includes index.
    1. Speech—Physiological aspects. 2. Hearing—Physiological aspects. 3. Anatomy,
Human. I. Title.
[DNLM: 1. Anatomy. 2. Speech—Physiology. 3. Hearing—Physiology.
WV 501 S359b]
QP306.S356    1984    612    83-26290


Croom Helm Ltd,
Provident House, Burrell Row
Beckenham, Kent BR3 1AT
England

ISBN 0-7099-3328-2

Printed in the United States of America

## Dedication

To my father, in loving memory.

# Preface

This text provides  a general introduction to anatomy  and physiology of the speech and  hearing mechanism,  primarily for  undergraduate college students.  Speech does not result from one isolated anatomical or physiological act,  or  from any obscure organ;  but rather,  by the dynamic activity of groups of specialized tissues.  To produce speech,  several systems are utilized.  The respiratory system generates the flow of air; the muscles modify structures via the nervous system; the nervous system orchestrates the whole.

   The subject matter in this text has been arranged to facilitate reading in connection with lecture and reference use.  After the first chapter, each chapter is arranged in four basic sections:

- Anatomy (skeletal and muscular systems, presented in outline form).

- Clinical considerations of physiology (function of the skeletal and muscular systems, presented in narrative form).

- Glossary of terms (supplementary to the terms used in the previous two sections).

- References (presentation of a variety of texts and journals, and citation of important contributions to the fields of speech, language, and hearing).


   Through this format,  it is hoped that the student  will acquire the foundation necessary to explore the subject more extensively.

viii

## Acknowledgments

Any success one achieves is due to the assistance and loyalty of others. The completion of this text is due in great measure to Susan for her patience and unyielding support, to Jeff and Angela for being themselves, to my parents for their constant guidance, and to R.L.M. who was the catalyst for my career choice.

My thanks also go to Jim Mitchell for his technical assistance with the manuscript, and to Jack Snowden for the graphics.

# CONTENTS

## FIGURES

# Chapter 1
# Introduction

## 1.1 Anatomical Landmarks

The human body is a complex and intricate structure that is examined from both an anatomical and a physiological perspective. The two views are not mutually exclusive. Anatomy is the science of the structure of organisms; physiology is the science of their function.

Anatomy is a descriptive science, and uses standardized terms. Names of structures usually describe their shape, or in the case of many muscles, are named for their origin and insertion. As a rule of thumb, the origin is considered the most fixed point, and the insertion is the most movable point. Occasionally, however, a structure may be named for a specific person. From the anatomical position which depicts the human figure standing, arms at the side, and palms of the hands forward, conventional terms are used to indicate planes or sections and locations throughout the body (Figure 1).

The Planes of the Body

1. SAGITTAL: a vertical cut from front to back.

2. CORONAL or FRONTAL: a vertical cut from side to side.

3. TRANSVERSE: a horizontal cut at any level.

General Terms of Location

1. VENTRAL: Away from the backbone.
   DORSAL: Toward the backbone.

2. ANTERIOR: Toward the front.
   POSTERIOR: Toward the back.

3. ROSTRAL: Toward the head.
   CAUDAL: Toward the tail.

4. SUPERIOR: Upper (toward the top).

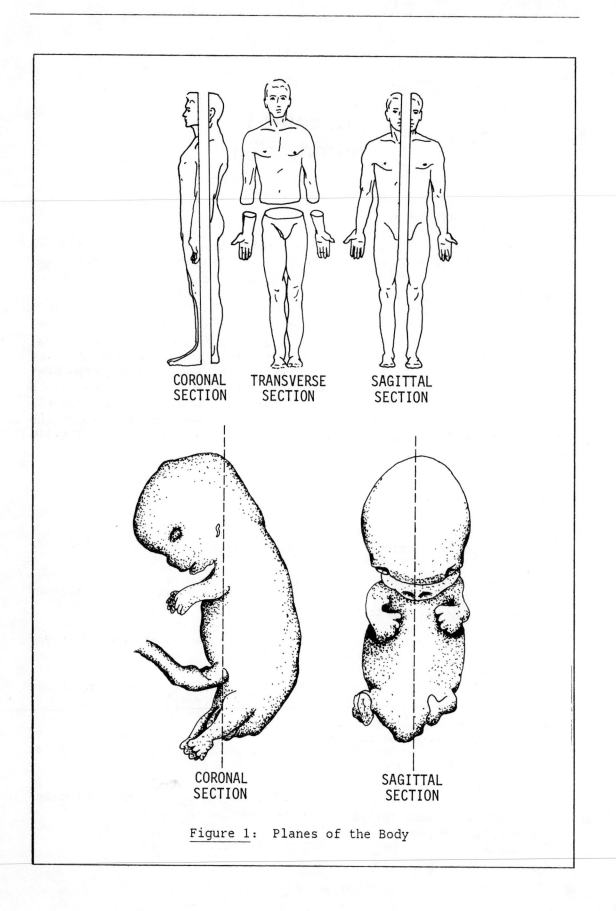

Figure 1:  Planes of the Body

INFERIOR: Lower (toward the tail).

5.  SUPERFICIAL: Toward the surface.
    DEEP: Away from the surface.

6.  EXTERNAL: Toward the outside.
    INTERNAL: Toward the inside.

7.  MEDIAL: Toward the axis, or near the midline.
    PERIPHERAL: Away from the axis or midline.
    LATERAL: Toward the side.

8.  PROXIMAL: Toward the axis or midline.
    DISTAL: Away from the axis or midline.

## General Principles of Multicellular Forms

The cell theory states that all animals and plants are composed of cells and cell products.  The cell is the fundamental unit of life, responsible for function of metabolism, reproduction, mobility, excretion, and response to stimuli.  In multicelluar forms, cells are organized for proper function; and, therefore, are differentiated both structurally and functionally.  A tissue is a group of cells of unique and similar structure and function.

1.  SUPPORTIVE tissue forms the scaffolding of the body.

    a.  BONE is inflexible and hard.

    b.  CARTILAGE is flexible and is softer than bone.  There are two types of cartilage.

        i.  HYALINE cartilage is dense and hard, and is found where rigidity is needed.

        ii.  ELASTIC cartilage is more flexible, and is found where protective cushioning is needed.

    c.  CONNECTIVE tissue holds cells together.  Its microscopic structure varies with the needs of the locality.

        i.  LIGAMENTS are tough, flexible strands and sheets of connective tissue which hold bones together at joints.

        ii.  TENDONS are tough, nonstretching links of connective tissue between muscles and bones.

2.  MUSCULAR tissue produces bodily movement.

a. There are three types of muscular tissues.

  i.   STRIATED (striped) muscles produce rapid "voluntary" motion such as required for speech.

  ii.  UNSTRIATED (smooth) muscle tissue produces slow, "involuntary" contractions. In human beings, it is found primarily in the viscera.

  iii. CARDIAC muscular tissue is capable of quick, rhythmic contractions, and of very prolonged periods of activity.

b. The action of muscle is to contract (shorten). Contraction of striated muscle exerts a pull upon the stuctures to which the muscle is attached.

c. To produce an opposite movement, another muscle (or muscles) pull(s) in the opposite direction. The opposed muscles are called ANTAGONISTIC, and their action is called ANTAGONISTIC MUSCLE ACTION.

  i.   FLEXOR muscles bend one part or another, as when biceps flex the forearm toward the upper arm.

  ii.  EXTENSOR muscles straighten or extend a part; triceps extend the forearm or upper arm.

  iii. ABDUCTOR draws a part away from the axis of the body; deltoid draws the arm forward.

  iv.  ADDUCTOR draws a part toward the axis of the body; latissimuss dorsi draws the arm up and back.

3. NERVE tissue, because of its extreme irritability and conductivity, is excited by changes either in the environment or within the body. It controls the muscular and glandular responses which are adjustments to these changes.

4. EPITHELIAL tissue forms the protecting and secreting covering of the external and internal body surfaces, cavities, and passageways.


General Principles of Organs

ORGANS are complex structures with functional unity.

• Each organ is a combination of several tissues.

• Each organ takes care of some essential body function (i.e. heart).

An ORGAN SYSTEM is a series of organs,  all of which have a part in performing a vital process essential to life (i.e.  digestive system).


## 1.2 Embryology

Study of  human development before birth  helps to understand  the relationships of normal  structures and potential causes  of congenital malformations.   Such conditions as cleft  palate and lip,  cerebral palsy, congenital malformation of arms,  legs,  and  ears may occur when normal development is interrupted.   Some causes of deviations present at birth are:

• Mutant genes.

• Chromosomal aberrations.

• Environmental teratogens (e.g. drugs like thalidomide).

• Multifactorial inheritance.


Development begins at conception ,when the sperm and egg unite.   The union forms a zygote,  which  immediately undergoes cell division.   The human EMBRYONIC period covers the time from conception until the seventh or eighth week.   Differentiation, or formation,  of body systems occurs during this period.   The eighth week until  birth is known as the FETAL period, and is a time primarily concerned with growth.   Throughout these developmental periods,   certain areas of the  embryo and fetus  grow at different rates.   The head region, for example, develops faster than the tail region (cephalocaudal development).

During the first four weeks of the embryonic period,  cellular layers are developing and differentiating  into specific anatomical structures. There are  three layers:  ECTODERM,  ENDODERM,  and a middle  layer of MESODERM.  From the outer ectoderm, the skin and nervous system evolves. The mesoderm develops into the  skeletal framework,  muscle,  connective tissue,  heart,  and blood  vessels.  The  innermost endodermal  layer becomes the respiratory and digestive systems.

The period between  the fourth and eighth weeks marks  the point when internal  and external  structures are  developed  to give  recognizable human characteristics.   By the beginning of the fourth week,  the branchial arches become  noticeable around the head and  neck region (Figure 2).   These  branchial arches  are six  ridges separated by grooves  or clefts.

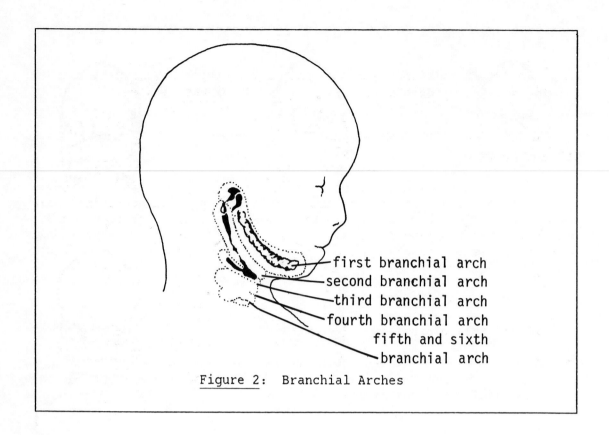

Figure 2:  Branchial Arches

The first branchial arch is involved with the development of the
face.   The dorsal portion of this arch,  known  as Meckel's cartilage,
forms two middle  ear bones called the MALLEUS and  INCUS.   The ventral
portion of the arch develops into the MANDIBLE, or lower jaw.   The second arch, aslo called Reichert's cartilage, forms the STAPES of the middle ear, the STYLOID process of the temporal bone of the skull, and portions of the  HYOID bone.   The third  arch forms the rest  of the hyoid
bone.   The fourth through sixth arches  form the cartilages of the larynx.

The  face develops  around  an opening  of the  embryo  known as  the
STOMODEUM, or primitive mouth.  Figure 3 illustrates the facial development that evolves around the stomodeum.    Superior to the mouth opening
is the FRONTONASAL PROCESS,  which will  become the forehead and part of
the nose.   Around the opening,  the portion of the first branchial arch
is developing into the MAXILLARY PROCESSES or upper jaw.  This branchial
arch is  also helping  to form  the lower  boundary of  the mouth:   the
MANDIBULAR PROCESS.   The paired mandibular processes grow to fuse anteriorly into a single unit by the fifth week.

Through the  fifth and seventh weeks,   the nasal region  develops to
form an INTERMAXILLARY SEGMENT of the upper jaw.  This segment forms the
mid portion of the upper lip, gingiva (gum ridge),  and the primary pal-

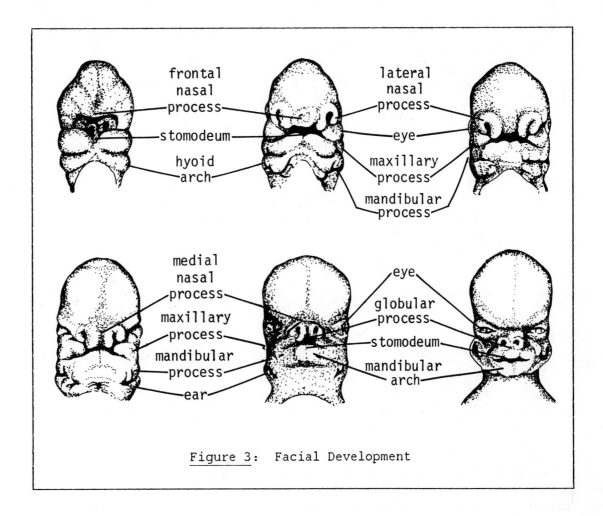

Figure 3:   Facial Development

ate.   The lateral parts  of the upper lip and the  secondary palate are
formed from the maxillary processes of the upper jaw.

   The series of pictures shown in  Figure 4 illustrate the palate (roof
of mouth) development.   As mentioned above,  the primary  palate is a
wedge-shaped structure developed from  the intermaxillary segment.   The
secondary palate develops from two projections of the maxillary process.
Projecting downward  between the tongue,  the processes  swing horizontally, meet, and fuse.   The secondary palate also fuses with the primary
palate  palate  and the nasal  septum.   Fusion of  the palate is  in an
anterior to  posterior direction (Figure 4),  and  is completed  by the
twelfth week  with the formation  of the  soft palate and uvula.   This
period marks the completion of the face.

   The eye is derived from aspects  of all cellular layers.   Again,  by
the fourth week,  optic grooves appear laterally on the embryo.   As the
facial region grows,  the eye region  moves medial to assume the characteristic position on  the face by the eighth week.   With this position

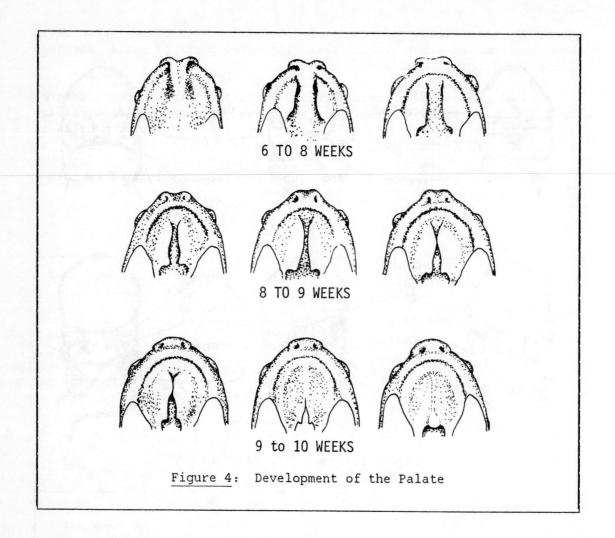

6 TO 8 WEEKS

8 TO 9 WEEKS

9 to 10 WEEKS

Figure 4:   Development of the Palate

change,   the eye developes its   intricate parts:   retina,   ciliary body,
iris, lens, etc.

    The ear develops into three regions:   external ear, middle ear,  and
inner ear.   The external ear develops  from the first branchial groove,
and forms the auricle and the auditory canal.   It is not until some time
in the fetal  period that the inner  part of the external  canal is complete.   The ear drum, or tympanic membrane, forms, separating the external ear from the middle ear.  As mentioned earlier, the ossicles (bones)
of the middle ear are from the  first and second branchial arches.   The
internal ear develops to form two structures:   the cochlea for hearing,
and the semicircular canals for balance.

    The respiratory system,  which includes the larynx and trachea,  also
begins to develop about the fourth  week.   The laryngeal cartilages and
muscles develop from the branchial arch cartilages,  and the vocal folds
develop from  folds of  membrane within  the larynx.   The lungs   first

appear at this time, and continue to develop even after birth until about the age of eight years, when the development of small air sacs within the lungs is complete.

Skeletal and muscle (myoblast cells) systems develop from mesoderm, first appearing in the fourth week, and developing as hyaline cartilage and bone. The skull, vertebral column, and ribs develop from cells in rostral, caudal, dorsal, and ventral directions.

The nervous system results from neural plates which later form into a neural tube (Figure 5).

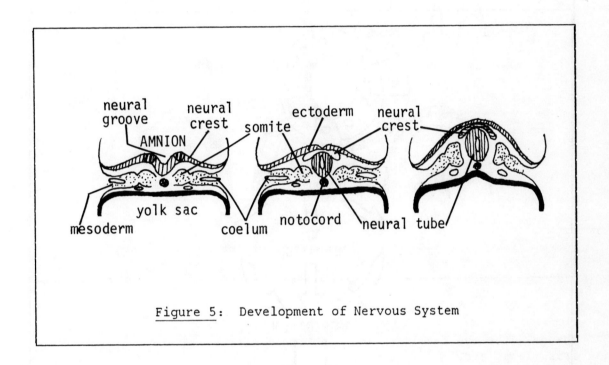

Figure 5:  Development of Nervous System

Cells at the edges of the neuroplate grow at a more accelerated rate than those cells at midline, and thus a neural groove is formed prior to formation of the neural tube. The rostral end of this tube becomes the brain, and the rest of the tube becomes the spinal cord; collectively called the CENTRAL NERVOUS SYSTEM. The PERIPHERAL NERVOUS SYSTEM which includes the spinal nerves, cranial nerves, and all other nervous tissue outside the central nervous system, is derived from the neural crest.

It is important for the introductory student to understand the embryological landmarks. It is also important to appreciate how these landmarks may have been formed. Three dynamic processes contribute to the development of anatomical regions: cell migration, merging, and fusion.

Illustrative of topographical change is the mesenchymal migration. At the risk of generalizing, it is sufficient to state that the mesenchyme cell becomes the mesodermal layer. Between the ectoderm and endoderm layers, the mesenchyme moves or migrates. MIGRATION begins by the cells freeing themselves of the bonds that hold them together. Why cells migrate, then reorganize, is still largely a mystery. But for some reason, cells of equal potentiality begin to bond together. This process is called AGGREGATION. From this aggregate state, cells multiply and differentiate, taking on recognizable characteristics (i.e., a blood vessel or vertebral primordium) ( Figure 6).

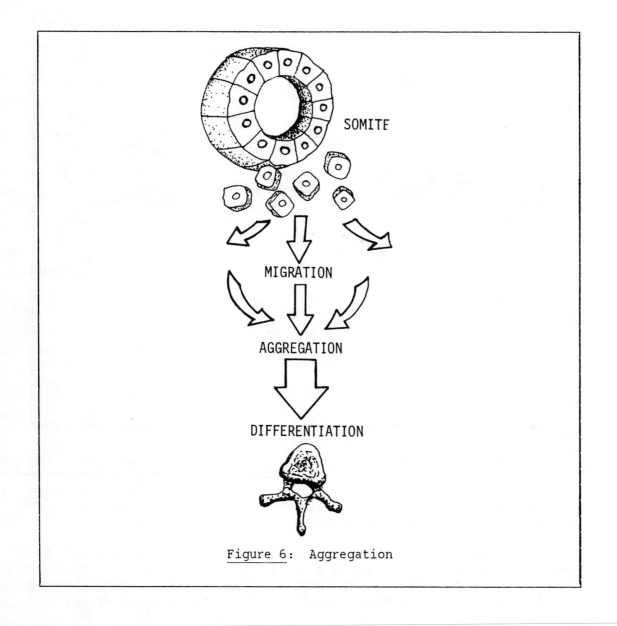

Figure 6:  Aggregation

Once mesenchymal growth takes place, originally paired structures such as the secondary palatal shelves of the maxillae join together by FUSION to form one functional unit. As shown in Figure 7, the two structures move together, and then the outer epithelial tissue layer dissolves and fusion is completed.

MERGING of tissue also accounts for regional changes, as cellular layers are "pushed" or extended to reach their intended configuration (Figure 7).

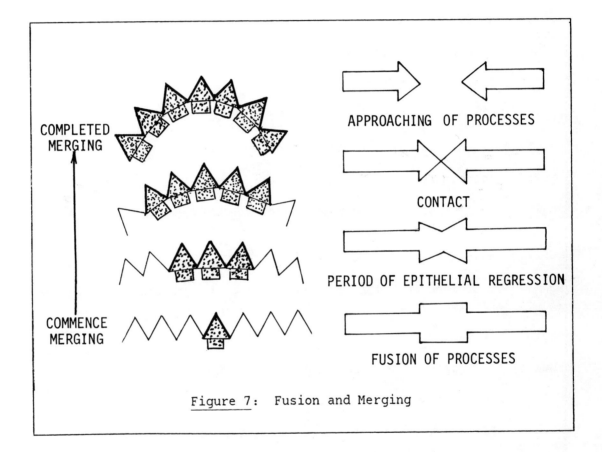

Figure 7:  Fusion and Merging

## 1.3 Anatomic Terms

aponeurosis:    Expanded tendon for the attachment of a flat muscle.

articulation:    Connection between bones.

belly:    Fleshy part of a muscle.

body:     Broadest or longest mass of a bone.

cartilage:     Substance from which some bone ossifies; gristle.

condyle:     Polished articular surface, usually rounded.

crest:     Ridge or border.

diaphysis:     The shaft of a long cylindrical bone.

eminence:     Low convexity just perceptible.

facet:     Small articular area, often a pit.

foramen:     Hole, perforation.

fossa:     Shallow depression.

head:     Enlarged round end of a long bone; knob.

insertion:     Relatively movable part of muscle attachment.

joint:     connection between bones.

ligament:     Fibrous tissue binding bones together, or holding tendons
     and muscles in place.

neck:     Constriction of a bone near head.

organ:     Two or more tissues grouped together to perform a highly spe-
     cialized function.

origin:     Relatively fixed part of a muscle attachment.

process:     Projection (can be grasped with fingers).

protuberance:     A swelling (can be felt under fingers).

ramus:     Platelike branch of a bone; branch of a vessel or nerve.

shaft:     Body of a long bone.

sheath:     Protective covering.

spine:     Pointed projection, or sharp ridge.

symphysis:     Union of right and left sides in the midline.

tendon:     Fibrous tissue securing a muscle to its attachment.

tubercle:    Small bump (can be felt under fingers).

tuberosity:    Large and conspicuous bump.


## 1.4 Terms for Direction and Movement

abduction (abd.):    Draws away from midline.

adduction (add.):    Draws toward the midline.

anatomic position:    Standing erect with arms at the sides and palms of
    the hands turned forward.

anterior (ant.) or ventral (vent.):    Situated before, or in front of.

corrugator:    That which wrinkles skin, draws skin in.

deep:    Farther from the surface (in a solid form).

depressor:    That which lowers.

distal (dist.):    Farther from the root.

dorsal (dors.) or posterior (post.):    Toward the rear, back; also back
    of hand, and top of foot.

erector:    That which draws upward.

extension (ext.):    Straightening.

external (extern.):    Outside (refers to wall of cavity or hollow
    form).

flexion (flex.):    Bending or angulation.

frontal (front.) or coronal (coron.):    Vertical; at right angles to
    sagittal; divides body into anterior and posterior parts.

inferior (inf.):    Lower, farther from crown of head.

lateral (lat.):    Farther from midline (or center plane).

levator (lev.):    That which raises.

medial (med.):    Nearer to midline (or center plane).

median:    Midway, being in the middle.

midline:    Divides body into a right and left side.

oblique:    Slanting.

posterior (post.) or dorsal (dors.):    Rear, or back.

proximal (prox.):    Nearer to limb root.

sagittal (sagit.):    Vertical plane or section dividing body into right and left portions.

sphincter:    That which regulates closing of aperture.

superficial (superf.):    Nearer to surface (refers to solid form).

superior (sup.):    Upper, nearer to crown of head.

tensor (tens.):    That which draws tight.

transverse (trans.):    At right angles to long axis; body divided into upper and lower parts.

ventral (vent.) or anterior (ant.):    situated before or in front of.


## 1.5 Embryonic Terms

amniocentesis:    Examination of amniotic fluid via fluid withdrawn from amniotic cavity; a tool in assessing potential disease to fetus.

conceptus:    Products of conception.

crown-rump length:    The "sitting" height measurement, used to determine length of embryo.

crown-heel length:    The "standing" height, used to measure length of fetus (after seven weeks).

fertilization age:    The reference point of 13 +/- 1 days, deducted from the menstrual age to obtain the actual age of an embryo.

genes:    The biological unit of heredity, located on a chromosome and transmitted from one generation to another.

mitosis:    The division of a cell.

placenta:    An organ attached to the uterus to join the mother and offspring during the embryologic and fetal periods.

postnatal:    Following birth.

prenatal:    Before birth.

somite:    Precursors of muscles and vertebrae.


## 1.6 Roots, Prefixes, and Suffixes

| | | |
|---|---|---|
| a-, (an-) | Greek | not; without |
| ab- | Latin | away from |
| acto- | Greek | tip or extremities; highest |
| ad- | Latin | toward |
| ambi- | Latin | both |
| amphi- | Greek | both; around |
| ana- | Latin | before |
| antero- | Latin | in front |
| anthrop- | Greek | human being; man |
| anti- | Greek | against |
| apo- | Greek | from; away from; off |
| arch- | Greek | first; chief; principal; great |
| aryten- | Greek | pitcher |
| auto- | Greek | self |
| bari- | Greek | heavy |
| bene- | Latin | well; good |
| bi- | Latin | two |
| biblio- | Greek | book |
| brachy- | Greek | abnormally short |
| brady- | Greek | slow |
| capit- | Latin | head |
| cardio- | Greek | heart |
| cata- | Greek | downward |
| cedi- | Latin | move; yield |
| centi- | Latin | hundred; hundredth |
| cephalo- | Greek | head |
| chrom- | Greek | color |
| chron- | Greek | time |
| circum- | Latin | round about |
| com- | Latin | with; together |
| contra- | Latin | against; in opposition |
| corp- | Latin | body |
| cresc- | Latin | rise; grow |
| crypto- | Greek | hidden; covered |
| cut- | Latin | skin |
| cycle- | Greek | ring; circle; cycle |
| de- | Latin | reversal; undoing |
| dec- | Greek | ten |
| demi- | Latin | half |
| dent- | Latin | tooth |
| derm- | Greek | skin |
| di- | Greek | twice |

| dia- | Greek | through; between; across |
| dic- | Latin | say |
| dis- | Latin | apart; separated from |
| dolicho- | Greek | long |
| duc- | Latin | lead |
| dyna- | Greek | power |
| dys- | Greek | ill; bad; hard |
| ec- | Greek | out of |
| ecto- | Greek | outside; external |
| -ectomy | Greek | surgical removal |
| embolo- | Greek | wedge; stopper |
| en- | Greek | in |
| endo- | Greek | inside |
| epi- | Greek | on; upon |
| eso- | Greek | inner |
| eu- | Greek | good; advantageous |
| ex- | Latin | out of; from |
| extero- | Latin | outside |
| extra- | Latin | beyond; outside of |
| fac- | Latin | make; do |
| fin- | Latin | end |
| flu- | Latin | flow |
| fort- | Latin | strong |
| gastro- | Greek | stomach |
| gen- | Greek | origin |
| glosso- | Greek | tongue |
| -gnosis | Greek | knowing; recognition |
| -gram | Greek | something drawn or written |
| -graph- | Greek | writing |
| helio- | Greek | sun |
| hemi- | Greek | half |
| hepta- | Greek | seven |
| hetero- | Greek | unlike; different |
| hexa- | Greek | six |
| histo- | Greek | tissue |
| homo- | Greek | same; similar |
| hydro- | Greek | water |
| hyper- | Greek | excess; over; superiority |
| hypno- | Greek | sleep |
| hypo- | Greek | under; inferior; less |
| idio- | Greek | personal; separate; distinct |
| infra- | Latin | below; lower |
| inter- | Latin | among; between; together |
| intro- | Latin | directed inward |
| -ism | Greek | state; condition |
| iso- | Greek | equal |
| -itis | Greek | inflammatory disease |
| juxta- | Latin | close to |
| kata- | Greek | downward (see cata-) |
| kilo- | Greek | thousand |
| kine- | Greek | movement |
| labio- | Latin | lip |

| | | |
|---|---|---|
| -lalia | Greek | speech |
| loc- | Latin | place |
| log- | Greek | words; reasoning |
| luc- | Latin | light |
| macro- | Greek | large |
| mal- | Latin | defect; bad |
| man- | Latin | hand |
| medio- | Latin | middle |
| mega- | Greek | great; powerful |
| meningo- | Greek | membrane |
| meso- | Greek | in the middle |
| meta- | Greek | after; change |
| -meter | Greek | measure |
| micro- | Greek | small |
| milli- | Latin | one thousandth; thousand |
| mis- | Latin | wrong |
| mono- | Greek | one; single |
| -morph | Greek | characterized by a specific form |
| multi- | Latin | many |
| myo- | Greek | muscle |
| neo- | Greek | new; recent |
| -nomy | Greek | a system of laws |
| non- | Latin | absence |
| oculo- | Latin | eye |
| -oid | Greek | like; resembling |
| -oma | Greek | growth; tumor |
| omni- | Latin | all |
| onto- | Greek | existing |
| -onym | Greek | name |
| -opia | Greek | relating to the eye |
| ortho- | Greek | straight; correct |
| -osis | Greek | diseased condition |
| oto- | Greek | ear |
| pan- | Greek | all |
| para- | Greek | faulty or disordered condition; subsidiary |
| -path | Greek | suffering |
| -pathy | Greek | feeling; disease; treatment |
| ped- | Latin | foot |
| pedo-, (ped-) | Greek | child |
| penta- | Greek | five |
| peri- | Greek | around |
| phil- | Greek | love |
| -phobia | Greek | morbid fear |
| phon- | Greek | sound |
| photo- | Greek | light |
| phren- | Greek | diaphragm; mind |
| pneumato- | Greek | air; respiration |
| pneumono- | Greek | lung |
| -pod | Greek | footed |
| poly- | Greek | many; manifold |
| post- | Latin | later; after |
| pre- | Latin | before |

| pro- | Latin | in front of; in place of |
| proto- | Greek | first in time or status |
| pseudo- | Greek | false; erroneous |
| psycho- | Greek | mind |
| pyro- | Greek | fire |
| quadr- | Latin | four |
| quasi- | Latin | seemingly |
| quinque- | Latin | five |
| re- | Latin | again |
| rect- | Latin | straight |
| ren- | Latin | kidney |
| retro- | Latin | backward; situated behind |
| rhino- | Greek | nose |
| -scope | Greek | instrument for observing |
| scoto- | Greek | darkness |
| -sect | Latin | cut; divided |
| semi- | Latin | half |
| sept- | Latin | seven |
| sex- | Latin | six |
| somno- | Latin | sleep |
| son- | Latin | sound |
| sphygmo- | Greek | pulse |
| spiro- | Latin | respiration |
| stereo- | Greek | a solid body |
| sub- | Latin | beneath; of lower order |
| super- | Latin | above; of higher order |
| supra- | Latin | above in position |
| syn- | Greek | together |
| tachy- | Greek | quick; swift |
| tele- | Greek | far |
| tetra- | Greek | four |
| thermo- | Greek | heat |
| thyro- | Greek | shield |
| -tomy | Greek | a cutting |
| trachy- | Greek | rough |
| trans- | Latin | across |
| tri- | Latin | three |
| ultra- | Latin | extreme; beyond |
| uni- | Latin | one |
| zo- | Greek | animal |

# References

Langman, J. (1969).  Medical embryology (2nd ed.).  Baltimore: Williams
    & Wilkins.

Moore, K. L. (1981).  Before we are born:  Basic embryology and birth
    defects (2nd ed.).  Philadelphia: Saunders Co.

Patten, B. M. (1968).  Human embryology (3rd ed.).  New York:
    McGraw-Hill.

Patten, B. M. (1971). Embryology of the palate and the maxillofacial
    region.  In W. C. Grabb, S. W. Rosenstein, & K. R. Bzoch (Eds.),
    Cleft lip and palate.  Boston: Little, Brown.

# Chapter 2
# Respiration

The respiratory system's  primary purpose is the exchange  of oxygen and
carbon dioxide to sustain life;  and secondarily, the provision of power
for phonation.   The flow of air from the lungs that generates the power
for voicing  results from muscle activity  of the abdomen,  chest,  and
back.   This chapter outlines the anatomy of respiration,  and discusses
the influence of these structures on phonation.

## 2.1 Skeletal System

Vertebral Column and Vertebrae

1.  The vertebral column is composed of 30 vertebrae that are grouped
    into five divisions (Figure 8).

    a.  CERVICAL vertebrae  form the  superior seven  vertebrae of
        the neck.

    b.  Twelve THORACIC vertebrae follow the cervical segment.

    c.  Five LUMBAR vertebrae succeed the thoracic portion.

    d.  The SACRUM,  a fairly broad  section,  is formed  by five
        fused vertebrae under the lumbar section.

    e.  The COCCYGEAL forms the most  inferior section of the col-
        umn,  and is composed of four small rudimentary vertebrae,
        considered together as one piece.

2.  A typical vertebra is made up of two main parts (Figure 9).

    a.  The CORPUS (body) is the largest part,  but varies in size
        from one vertebral division to another.

    b.  The VERTEBRAL ARCH consists of pedicles, laminae, and pro-
        cesses.  A vertebra has three characteristic processes.

i.   ARTICULAR processes extend upward and downward, and
     articulate with adjacent vertebrae.

ii.  SPINOUS processes are directed dorsally from the
     lamina.

iii. TRANSVERSE processes project laterally between the
     superior and inferior articular facet at approxi-
     mately the mid-region of the vertebrae.

3.  The joint between the vertebrae is composed of a cartilaginous
    INTERVERTEBRAL DISC and a complex bond of ligaments.

    a.  The intervertebral discs absorb shock to the vertebral
        column.

    b.  One-fourth of the length of the vertebral column is com-
        posed of the discs.

4.  There are four movements of the vertebral column:

    a.  FLEXION is bending forward.

    b.  EXTENSION is bending backward.

    c.  LATERAL FLEXION is bending side to side.

    d.  ROTATION represents twisting of the trunk.

## Ribs

1.  There are 12 pairs of ribs.  Each rib can be divided into three
    regions (Figure 10).

    a.  The vertebral attachment is the point of articulation for
        the rib and the vertebra.

    b.  The corpus, or body of the rib, is the longest segment of
        the rib.

    c.  The sternum is the ventral portion of the rib.

2.  The first seven pairs of ribs are collectively classified as
    VERTEBROCOSTAL.  They each articulate dorsally with the verte-
    brae; and ventrally, via hyaline costal cartilage, with the ster-
    num.

3.  The lowest four pairs of ribs are classified as FALSE ribs.

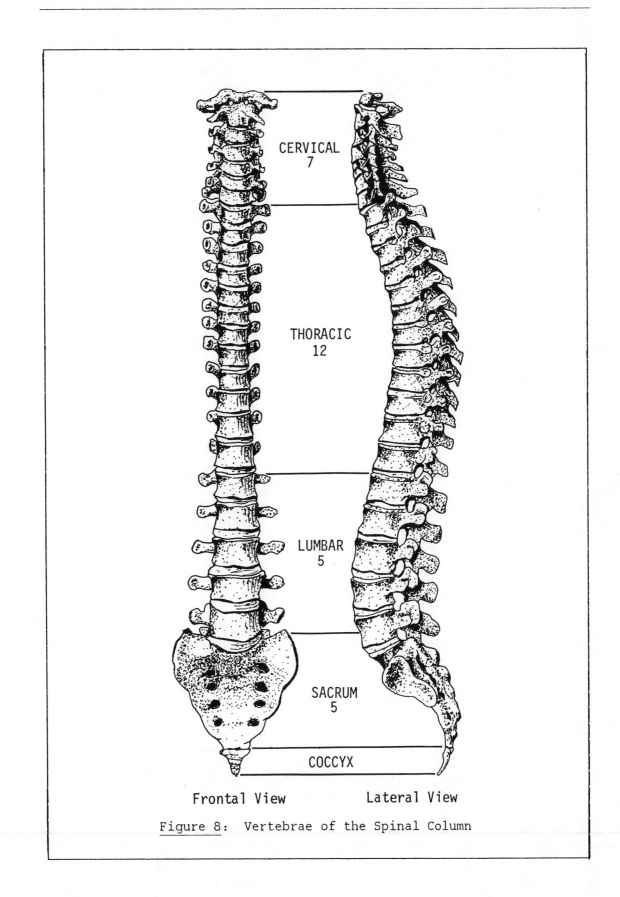

CERVICAL
7

THORACIC
12

LUMBAR
5

SACRUM
5

COCCYX

Frontal View          Lateral View

Figure 8:  Vertebrae of the Spinal Column

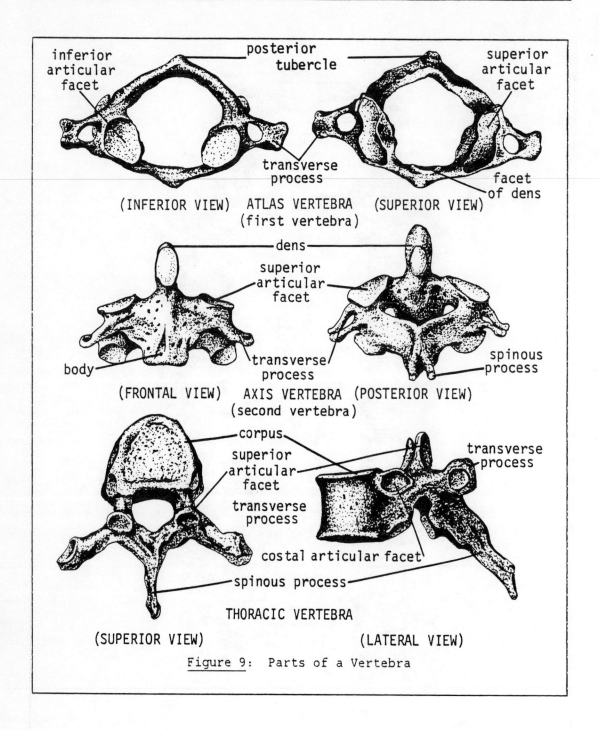

Figure 9:  Parts of a Vertebra

a.  Ribs 8 to 10 differ from the ribs above by ventrally joining in a common costal cartilage, giving them indirect attachment to the sternum.

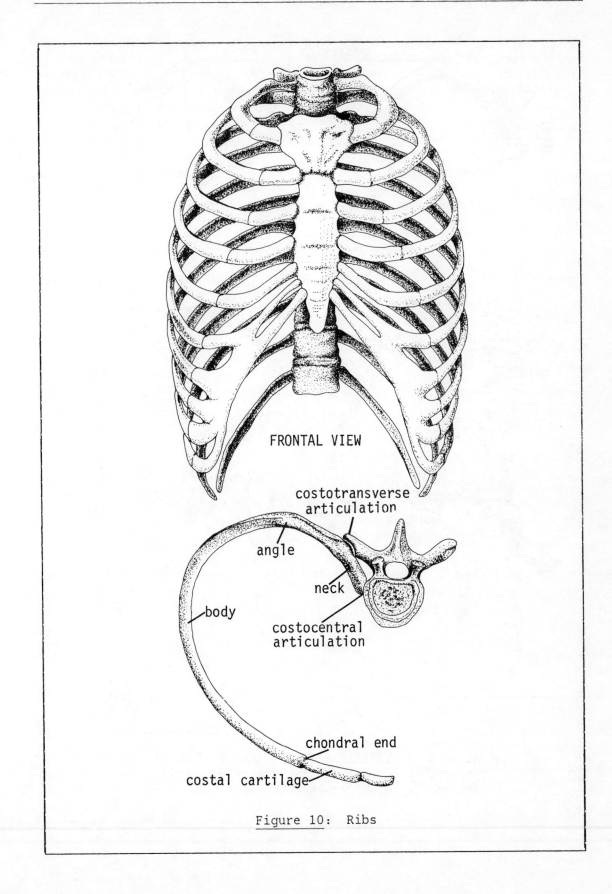

FRONTAL VIEW

costotransverse
articulation

angle

neck

body

costocentral
articulation

chondral end

costal cartilage

Figure 10:  Ribs

b.  Ribs 11 and 12 are free at the ventral end, and are embedded in abdominal muscle.

4.  Movement of the ribs resulting during inspiration is in an upward
direction.  Because the curve of each rib is greater than the one
above, the diameter of thorax increases, allowing air to be taken
into the lungs.

Sternum

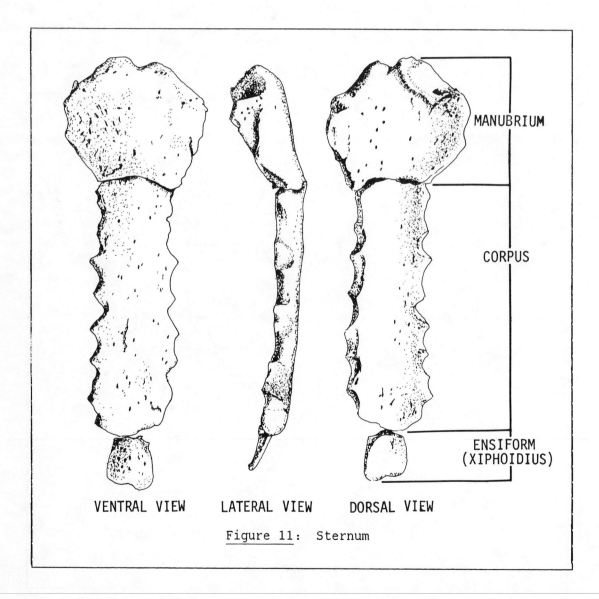

VENTRAL VIEW      LATERAL VIEW      DORSAL VIEW

Figure 11:  Sternum

1.  The sternum is an oblong plate located ventrally, and is composed
    of three areas (Figure 11).

    a.  The MANUBRIUM is the upper part.

    b.  The CORPUS is the central and largest section.

    c.  The ENSIFORM  (xiphoideus)  is an  inferior cartilagenoric
        portion.

2.  The upper seven or eight pairs of ribs have their cartilages fas-
    tened directly to the sternum.

3.  The sternum moves upward and forward during inspiration.

Coxal Bone

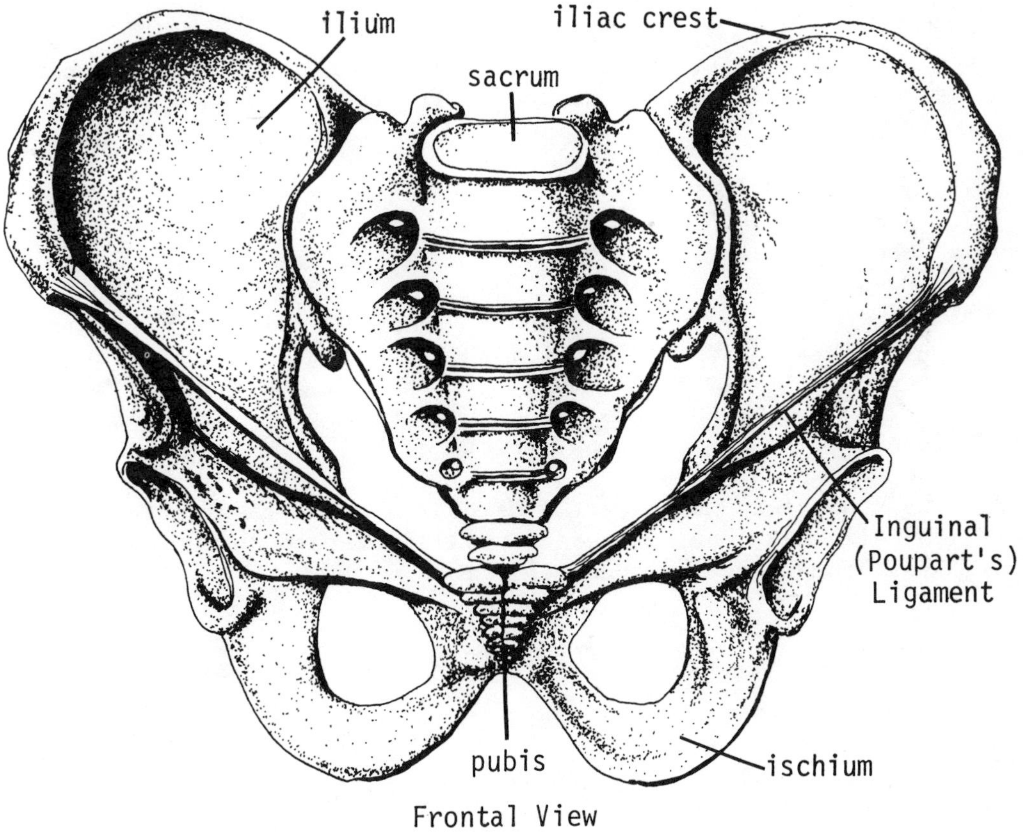

Figure 12:  Coxal Bone

1.  The coxal bone is paired, forming most of the pelvis (Figure 12). This bone is composed of three parts.

    a.  The ILIUM is the broad upper portion of the hip.

    b.  The ISCHIUM is the inferior portion of the bone.

    c.  The PUBIS is the most inferior medial segment.

2.  Posteriorly, the coxal bone articulates with the sacrum of the vertebral column. Anteriorly, the pubic areas project medially and join at the pubic symphysis.

## Clavicle (collar bone)

1.  The CLAVICLE is situated anteriorly and superiorly to the sternal end of the first rib (Figure 13). It attaches medially to the manubrium of the sternum, and attaches laterally to the scapula.

2.  The two clavicles function primarily to support the arm; however, several muscles which attach to it may influence the ribs for breathing.

## Scapula (shoulder blade)

1.  The scapula is a triangular shaped bone (Figure 13, right panel) located dorsally to the upper eight ribs. Laterally, it attaches to the clavicle in the shoulder girdle region. Medially, the bone is not attached to a bony structure.

2.  The scapula is not directly responsible for respiration, but like the clavicle, has several muscles attached which can influence breathing by pulling upon the ribs.

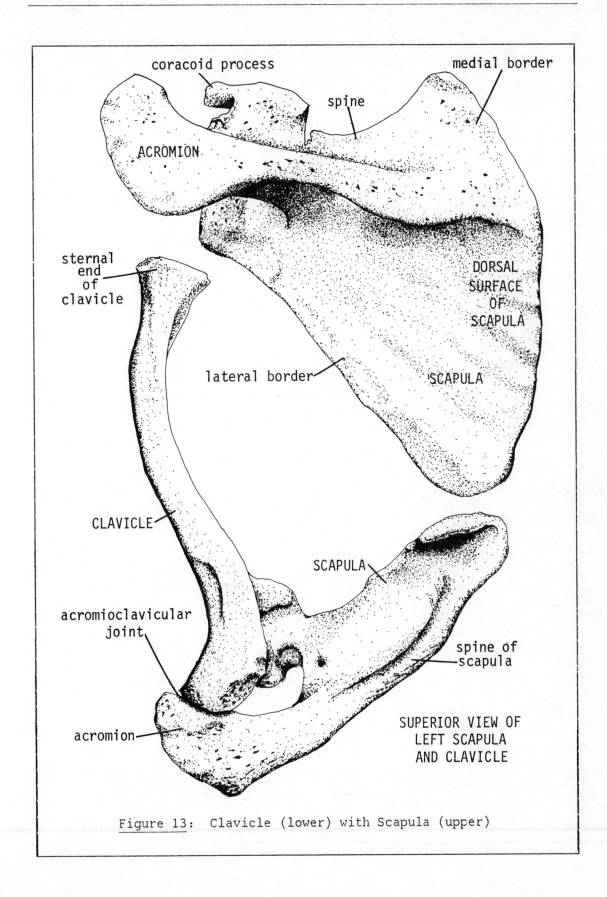

coracoid process

medial border

spine

ACROMION

sternal
end
of
clavicle

DORSAL
SURFACE
OF
SCAPULA

lateral border

SCAPULA

CLAVICLE

SCAPULA

acromioclavicular
joint

spine of
scapula

acromion

SUPERIOR VIEW OF
LEFT SCAPULA
AND CLAVICLE

Figure 13:  Clavicle (lower) with Scapula (upper)

## 2.2 Muscular System

<u>The Abdominal Muscles</u>

1.  The lateral abdominal wall contains three layers of muscle.

    a.  The EXTERNAL OBLIQUE (paired) (Figure 14) is the strongest
        and most superficial of the abdominal wall.

        i.   The muscle rises  from the inferior borders  of the
             lower eight ribs,  and interdigitates with the pec-
             toralis major,  serratus  anterior,  and latissimus
             dorsimus.

        ii.  Its fibers have a three-fold insertion.

             1) Most of the fibers  join the most superficial
                layer of the abdominal aponeurosis, a tendon
                which is usually flat, broad, and sheetlike.

             2) Inferior to these are fibers attaching to the
                INGUINAL (Poupart's) ligament.

             3) The lowest  and most posterior  fibers insert
                along the iliac crest.

    b.  The INTERNAL OBLIQUE muscle (paired)  (Figure 14)  is deep
        to the external oblique.

        i.   This muscle rises from three points of origin.

             1) The dorsal  inferior attachment  is from  the
                band or  sheet of fibrous  connective tissue
                called the lumbar FASCIA.

             2) The  inferior-lateral  attachment is  on  the
                iliac crest (hip bone).

             3) The  inferior-ventral  origin  is  along  the
                INGUINAL ligament.

        ii.  Its fibers  course primarily upward to  insert into
             three distinct regions.

             1) The uppermost fibers go  to the cartilages of
                ribs 10, 11, and 12.

2) The main mass of fibers  attach to the middle
sheet of the ABDOMINAL aponeurosis.

3) The inferior fibers attach to the pubis.

c.  The TRANSVERSE ABDOMINAL muscle  (paired)  (Figure 15)  is
deep to the internal oblique muscles.

i.  The  muscle originates  from  the  surfaces of  the
lower ribs (6),  from the  lumbar fascia,  from the
iliac crest, and from Poupart's ligament.

ii.  Its fibers run horizontally.

1) Most  insert into  the deepest  layer of  the
abdominal aponeurosis.

2) A few fibers attach to the pubis, and to Poupart's ligament.

2.  The  ventral abdominal  wall is  formed by  the narrow  segmented
RECTUS muscle (paired) (Figure 15).

a.  This muscle parallels the midline,   bisected by the linea
alba.

b.  It originates superiorly at the xiphoid process and costal
cartilages 5, 6, and 7.

c.  The point of insertion is at the pubis.

d.  The  upper two-thirds  of the  rectus are  encased by  the
abdominal aponeurosis,  while  the lower third is  deep to
it.

Diaphragm

The DIAPHRAGM (single) is an arched musculo-tendonous partition dividing
the thoracic and abdominal cavities (Figure 16).

1.  It consists of muscle fibers which arch upward to become continuous with a  central aponeurotic tendon in the center  of the dia-
phram.

2.  It is divided into three parts.

a.  The VERTEBRAL  portion has  its origin  on the  upper four
lumbar vertebrae.

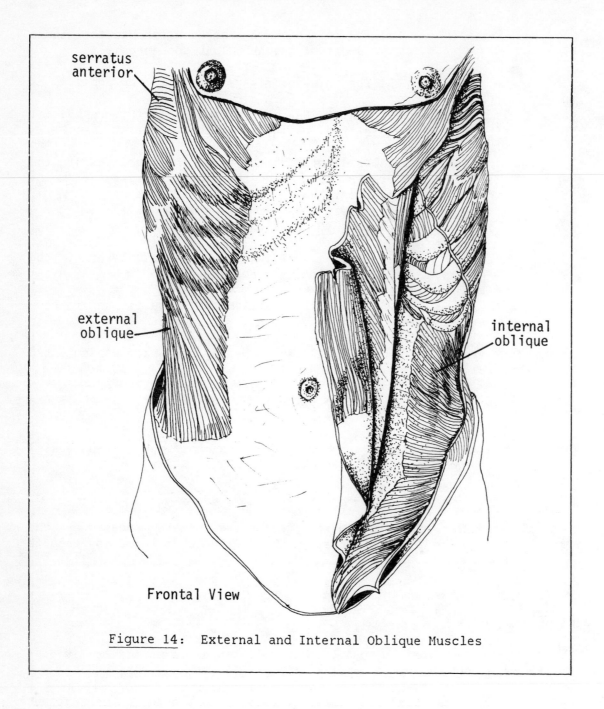

Figure 14:  External and Internal Oblique Muscles

    b.  The COSTAL  portion (paired)  rises from  the lowest  six ribs, and from their cartilages.

    c.  The STERNAL  portion originates on  the dorsal  surface of the xiphoid process.

3.  The muscle fibers insert at the CENTRAL TENDON.

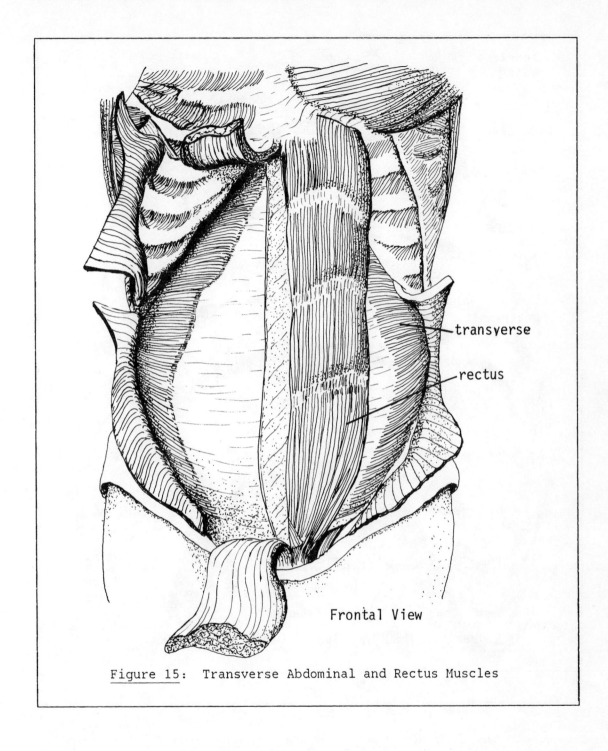

transverse

rectus

Frontal View

Figure 15:  Transverse Abdominal and Rectus Muscles

4.  Upon contraction,  the diaphragm flattens,  enlarging  the chest
    cavity, and displacing the abdominal viscera.

The diaphragm is pierced by nerves,  blood vessels,  and the alimentary
tract.  There are three major openings in the diaphragm.

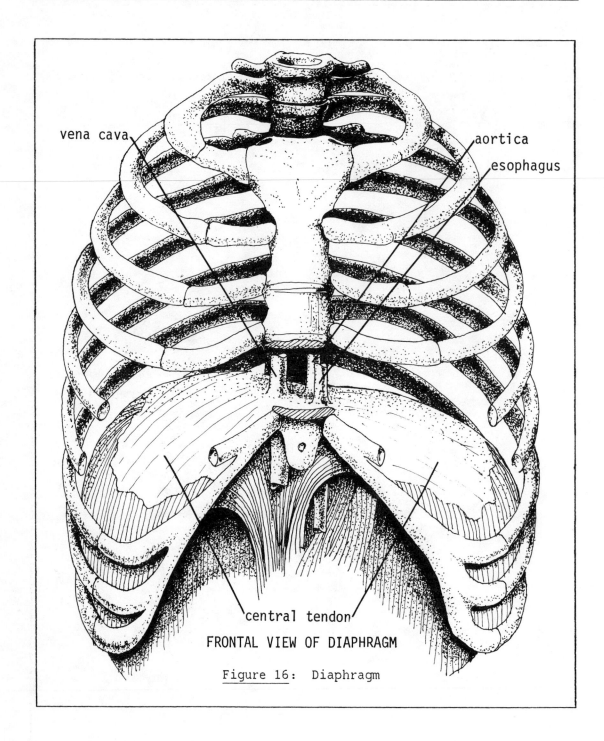

FRONTAL VIEW OF DIAPHRAGM

Figure 16:  Diaphragm

1.  The HIATUS AORTICUS is near the vertebral column.

2.  The HIATUS ESOPHAGEUS is near the central tendon.

3.  The FORAMEN VENAE CAVA is in the central tendon.

Muscles of the Chest, Neck, and Back

The CHEST MUSCLES influence rib position during respiration (Figure 17).

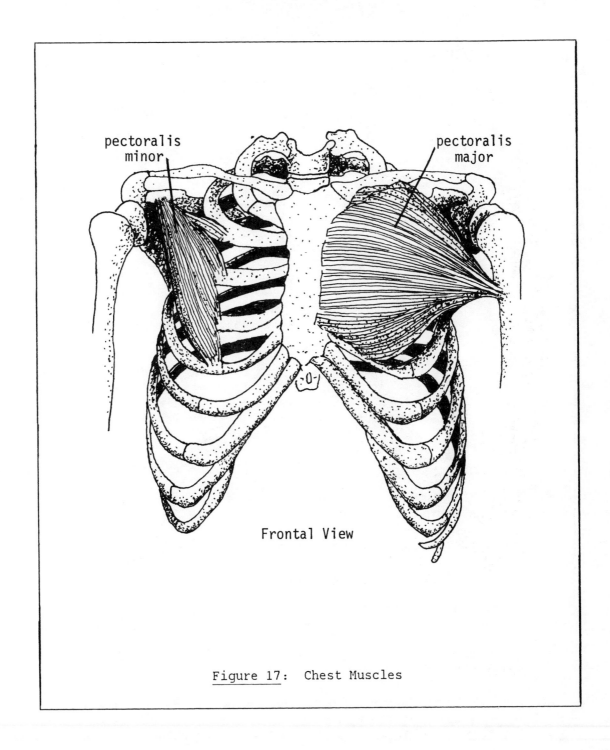

Figure 17:  Chest Muscles

1.  The PECTORALIS MAJOR (paired) is on the superficial surface of the anterior thoracic wall (Figure 17).

    a.  They originate from the clavical, sternum, costal cartilages 2-7, and the superficial layer of the abdominal aponeurosis.

    b.  Their fibers run to the side, inserting at the promixal part of the humerus.

    c.  The pectoralis major aids in raising the ribs for inspiration.

2.  The PECTORALIS MINOR (paired) is deep to the pectoralis major (Figure 17).

    a.  They originate from the surface of the second through the fifth ribs.

    b.  Their fibers insert by tendon at the coracoid process of the scapula.

    c.  These muscles help raise the ribs for inspiration.

3.  The SERRATUS ANTERIOR (paired) is on the lateral-posterior wall of the thorax (Figure 14).

    a.  These muscles originate from the upper eight or nine ribs.

    b.  Their fibers curve sideward and backward to insertion on the scapula.

    c.  The serratus anterior aids in raising the ribs during inspiration.

4.  The SUBCLAVIUS (paired) are short muscles between the clavicle and the first rib.

    a.  They originate from the first rib.

    b.  They insert on the clavicle.

    c.  These muscles draw the first rib upward during respiration.

5.  The EXTERNAL INTERCOSTALS (paired) are thin fibers sitting in the intercostal spaces (Figure 18).

    a.  The fibers rise from the lower margin of one rib and insert at the upper margin of the rib below.

b.  They extend from the vertebral column to the costal cartilages.

c.  They eliminate the alternate bulging out and sucking in of intercostal tissue during breathing.

6.  The INTERNAL INTERCOSTALS lie deep to the external intercostals.

a.  They rise from the lower margin of each rib, and insert on the upper margin of the rib below (Figure 18).

b.  They extend from the sternum to points a short distance from the vertebral column.

c.  The muscles help to eliminate collapse of the intercostal walls.

7.  The TRANSVERSE THORACIS (Triangularis sterni) (paired) are on the posterior surface of the anterior thoracic wall.

a.  These muscles rise from the corpus sterni and xiphoid process (Figure 19).

b.  The fibers run upward to the side and insert along the posterior surfaces of the third through the sixth costal cartilages.

c.  They reinforce the intercostals.

8.  The SUBCOSTALS (paired) lie on the ventral surface of the dorso-lateral thoracic wall.

a.  They parallel and are deep to the internal intercostals.

b.  The subcostals vary in number and detail.

c.  They originate lateral to the vertebrae, on the inner surface of the ribs.

d.  They insert on the deep surface of the second or third rib above the point of origin.

e.  The subcostals maintain relative positions of ribs.

## Neck Muscles that Influence Rib Position

Two neck muscles influence rib position for respiration (Figure 20).

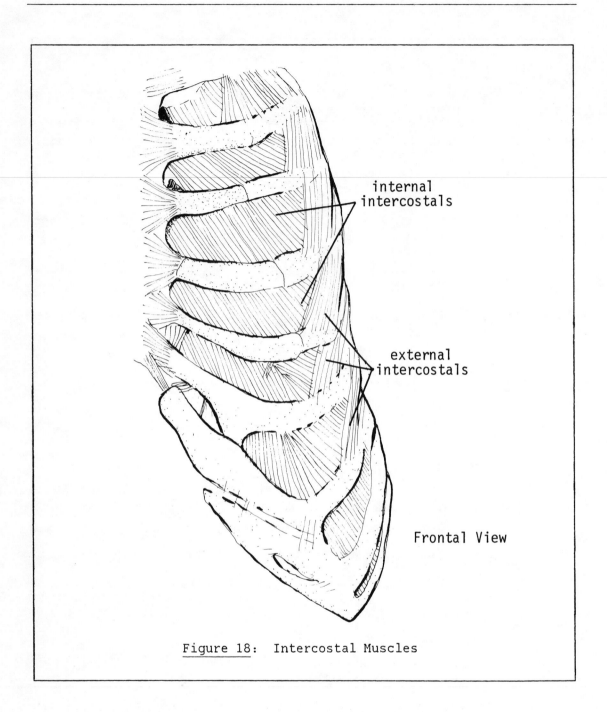

Figure 18:   Intercostal Muscles

1.  The STERNOCLEIDOMASTOID  (paired)  are strong muscles  which pass
    upward and lateralward across the side of the neck.

    a.  They are divided into two heads.

        i.  The STERNAL HEAD rises from the manubrium sterni.

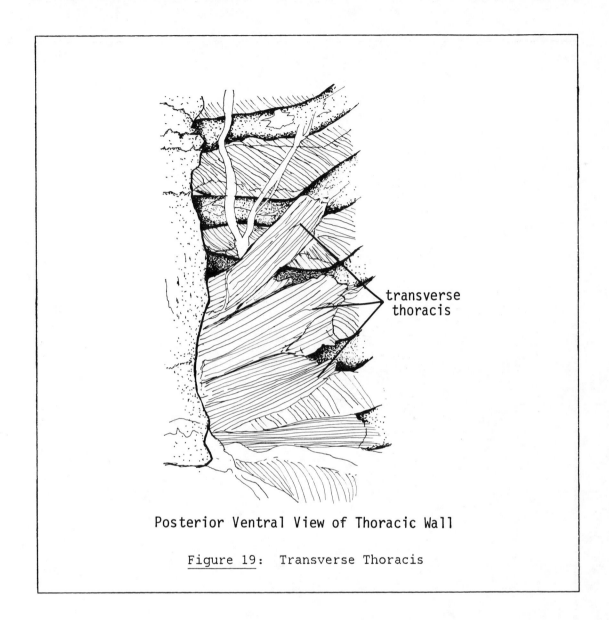

Posterior Ventral View of Thoracic Wall

Figure 19:   Transverse Thoracis

        ii.   The CLAVICULAR  HEAD originates on the  sternal end
           of the clavicle.

   b.   The two heads  unite before inserting on  the lateral sur-
      face of the mastoid.

   c.   These muscles raise the sternum,  and indirectly the ribs,
      during inspiration.

2.   The SCALENI form a triangular muscle group located in the lateral
   part of the neck.

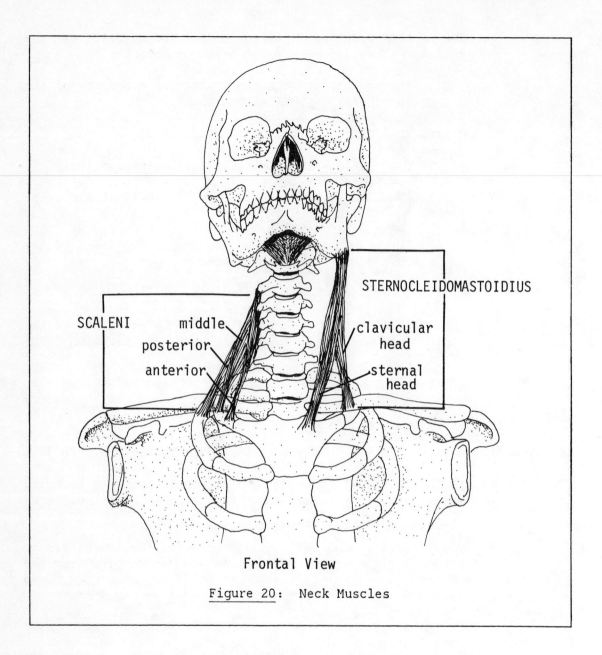

Frontal View

Figure 20:  Neck Muscles

a. The SCALENUS ANTERIOR (paired) are deep to the sternocleidomastoid.

   i.   They originate  on the transverse processes  of the third through sixth cervical vertebrae.

   ii.  The fibers insert on the first rib.

   iii. These muscles elevate the first rib during inspiration.

b.  The SCALENUS MEDIUS (paired)   are  the longest  of  the scaleni.  They lie behind the scalenus anterior.

    i.  They originate from the transverse processes of the six INFERIOR CERVICAL VERTEBRAE.

    ii.  They insert on the FIRST RIB.

    iii.  They elevate the first rib during inspiration.

c.  The SCALENUS POSTERIOR (paired) are the smallest and deepest of the scaleni.

    i.  The origin is from the  transverse processes of the lower three cervical vertebrae.

    ii.  They insert on the second rib.

d.  The SCALENI  muscle group influences  the position  of the sternum and the  other true ribs during  inspiration (Figures 20 and 21).

## Back Muscles Affecting Respiration

Certain back muscles affect both inspiration and expiration (Figure 21).

1.  The LATISSIMUS DORSIMUS (paired)  are triangular muscles covering the dorso-lateral area of the lumbar and lower half of the thoracic regions.

a.  They rise from the spinous processes  of the lowest six or seven thoracic vertebrae, from the lumbar fascia, from the external surfaces of  the lowest three or  four ribs,  and from the iliac crest.

b.  The fibers converge upward and lateralward, to attach by a long tendon to the humerus.

c.  These muscles may raise the lowest three or four ribs.

2.  The SERRATUS POSTERIOR SUPERIOR (paired) are located on the outer surface of the dorsal part of the upper thoracic wall.

a.  Their origin is  by a broad tendon from the  lowest one or two cervical and upper two or three thoracic vertebrae.

b.  The fibers  of these  muscles insert  just beyond  the rib angles.

3.  The SERRATUS POSTERIOR INFERIOR (paired)   lie on the dorsal wall
    at the lumbar and thoracic regions.

    a.  They rise from the spinous  process of the lowest thoracic
        and upper lumbar vertebrae (Figure 21).

    b.  Their fibers insert just beyond the rib angles on the four
        lowest ribs.

    c.  These muscles may draw the  lowest four ribs downward dur-
        ing exhalation.

4.  The vertebral column is flanked on  either side by a complex mass
    of muscles, the SACROSPINALIS (paired), whose main function is to
    produce movements of the vertebral  column.   Parts of these mus-
    cles may influence rib movement.

    a.  The ILIOCOSTALIS LUMBORUM (paired) depress the ribs during
        **ex**halation.

    b.  The ILIOCOSTALIS  DORSI (paired)  are  a series  of narrow
        muscles  which  bind  the ribs,   allowing  them  to  move
        together during exhalation.

    c.  The ILIOCOSTALIS CERVICIS (paired) elevate the ribs during
        inspiration.

5.  The COSTAL ELEVATORS (paired)  lie immediately to the side of the
    vertebral column (Figure 21).

    a.  They rise from the transverse processes of the lowest cer-
        vical and upper thoracic vertebrae.

    b.  They  are divided  into two  groups,   according to  their
        insertions.

        i.   The LEVATORES  COSTARUM BREVIS  inserts to  the rib
             immediately below its origin.

        ii.  The LEVATORES COSTARUM LONGE  inserts on the second
             rib below its origin.

    c.  These muscles may aid in  raising these ribs during inspi-
        ration.

6.  The QUADRATUS  LUMBORUM (paired)  are  located within  the dorsal
    abdominal wall (Figure 21).

    a.  These muscles originate  along the iliac crest  and lumbar
        ligaments.

b.  They insert on the twelfth rib and the transverse processes of the upper lumbar vertebrae.

c.  The quadratus lumborum draws the last rib down and anchors it against the pull of the diaphragm during respiration.

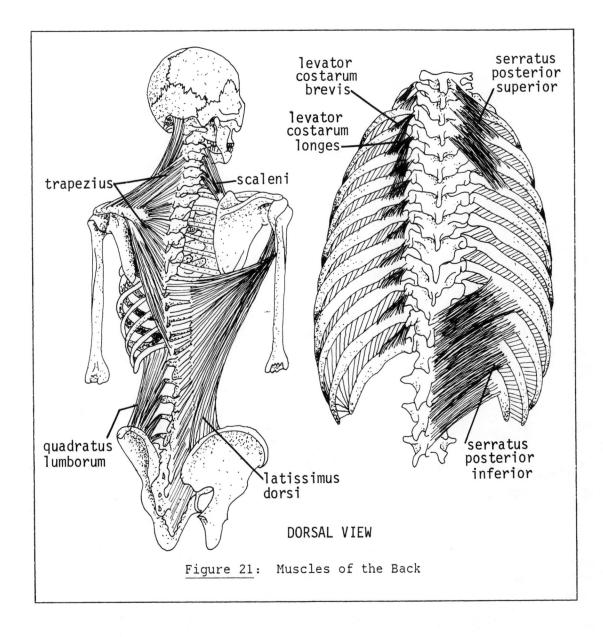

DORSAL VIEW

Figure 21:  Muscles of the Back

Lungs

The LUNGS are two roughly conical  masses of spongy material composed of minute  air cells  (Figure 22).   They  are  the  site  where the  blood receives oxygen and gives off carbon dioxide (Figure 24).

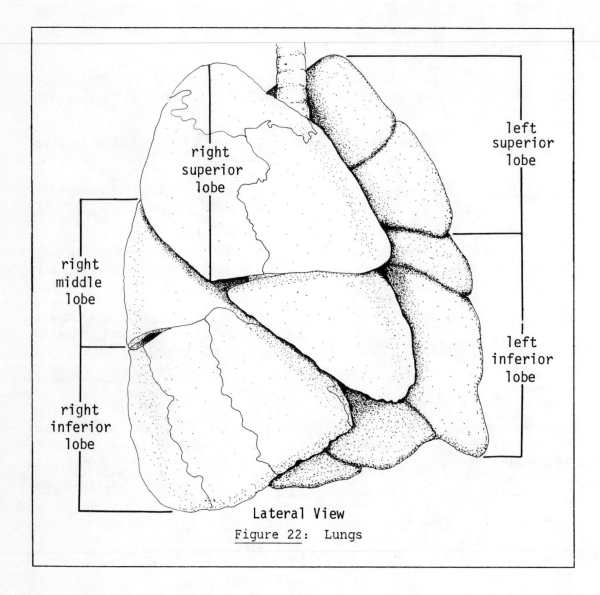

Lateral View

Figure 22:  Lungs

1.  The TRACHEA  is an elastic tube  through which air passes  to and from the lungs.

    a.  It is a  midline structure situated in the  neck and upper chest regions.

b.  It is composed of horseshoe-shaped hyaline cartilages connected by membrane.  The posterior wall of the trachea is membranous.

2.  At its lower end the trachea bifurcates  to give rise to two MAIN STEM BRONCHI.

3.  The lungs are  fastened only by the bronchi to  the trachea.  At all other places  they are against the walls of  the thorax,  but are not attached thereto.

4.  Each main stem  bronchus gives off branches which  in turn subdivide repeatedly.  The narrowest tubular  branches of this system are the BRONCHIOLI.

a.  The bronchioli are found in all parts of the lungs (Figure 23).

b.  The bronchioli  divide to give  rise to  DUCTULI AVEOLARES which in  turn communicate  with air  sacs called  SACCULI AVEOLARES.

c.  The walls of the sacculi aveolares, and to a lesser extent those of the ductuli and  bronchioli,  are pitted with air cells called ALVEOLI (Figure 24).

i.  The lung  contains about 14 million  alveolar ducts which give rise to  approximately 300 million alveoli.

ii.  The walls of  the alveoli are thin  membranes which are rich in capillaries.

The PLURAE are  two lubricated SEROUS MEMBRANES.  One  covers the lungs and the other lines the inner surface of the thoracic wall.  They form a double layer between lungs and body wall called the pleural linkage.

1.  VISCERAL PLEURA surround the lung.

2.  PARIETAL PLEURA surround the surface of the thorax.

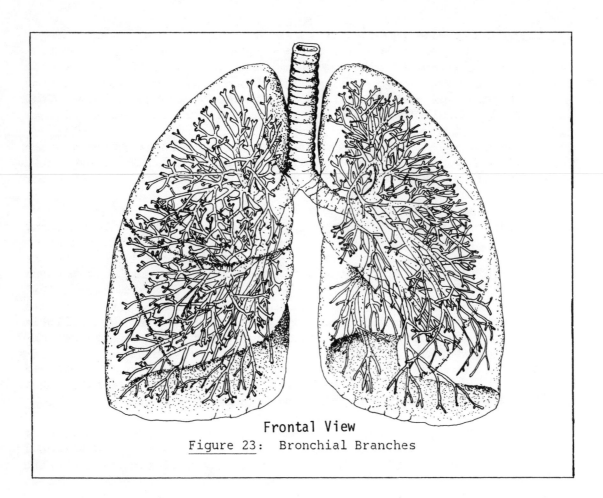

Frontal View

Figure 23:  Bronchial Branches

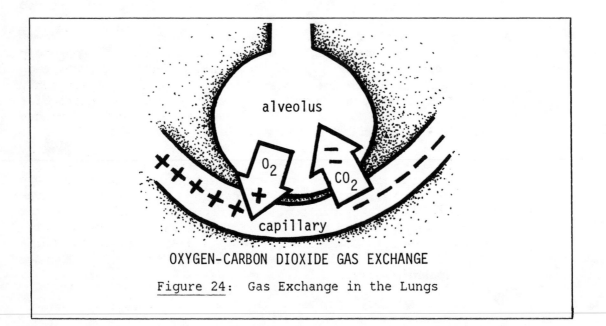

OXYGEN-CARBON DIOXIDE GAS EXCHANGE

Figure 24:  Gas Exchange in the Lungs

## 2.3 Mechanics of Breathing

The foremost purpose of  respiration is to supply the cells  of the body
with needed oxygen,  and to remove carbon dioxide.   This task is accomplished by the combined efforts  of the pulmonary,  cardiovascular,  and
the neural systems.  The structures necessary for respiration serve secondarily in humans to produce a  controlled air stream which,  modified,
results in speech.   The physical  and mechanical aspects of respiration
can be  studied as they relate  to the basic biological  functions (i.e.
vegetative or  tidal breathing),  and as  they contribute to  speech and
language.

   Vegetative breathing to sustain life  is accomplished by the movement
of air in and out of the lungs.  Air enters the lungs when the intrathoracic pressure is  lowered .   Air is  forced out of the  lungs when the
intrathoracic pressure is increased.   The inspiratory muscles are those
that run from the head,  neck,  shoulder girdle to the ribs;  those that
run from rib to rib (downward and  inward);  and those back muscles that
run from the  cervical and thoracic vertebrae to  the ribs (triangularis
sterni).   Because of the  shape of the ribs and their  angle of attachment, there is an outward rotation as the rib is pulled upward,  resulting in an increased size of the  thoracic cavity.  The lung follows the
movement of the chest wall.   Three-fourths  of the lung's surface makes
contact with the thoracic wall via the pleural linkage.

   Expiration begins when gravitational forces and the elastic nature of
the expanded lung  and chest tissue are allowed to  recoil.   The recoil
raises the pressure within the lungs to exceed atmospheric pressure, and
air is expelled from the lungs.   For greater expiratory effort such as
required  in exercise  and speech,  accessory muscles  come into  play.
Expiratory muscles are those that run from  the pelvis to the sternum or
ribs; or from the vertebrae upward to the ribs; rib to rib (downward and
outward); and from the sternum.

   During speech production significant changes occur in the respiratory
cycle from that observed in vegetative breathing.   Breathing for speech
involves  a controlled  prolonged  expiration  with rapid  inspirations.
During conversational  speech the abdominal  muscles are  contracted for
both expiration  and inspiration.   This mechanical  maneuver influences
the action of the diaphragm.

   During expiration, the chest and abdominal walls actively control the
breath stream.   The diaphragm moves upward,  and the costal fibers are
stretched,  resulting in  their ability to respond  quickly for inspiration.   The diaphragm quickly contracts to overcome the influence of the
chest wall;  but the abdominal muscles remain taut and the ribs are elevated.  The result of this complex adjustment is almost continuous unin-
terrupted flow of speech.   Without such a maneuver, our speech-language
would be slowed considerably.

To sustain a  steady level of phonation  for a long time,   the lungs
decrease in volume.    This respiratory action is  necessary to maintain
subglottic air  pressure and glottal air  flow (the glottis is  the area
between the vocal folds).  Expiration for speech is different from expiration for sustained phonation because during conversation intensity and
pitch changes occur continually throughout the utterance.

Lung volume  levels used in  connected speech increase  when loudness
varies.    Loudness, however,  in connected speech is the result of both
respiratory and laryngeal changes.  The net effect is higher lung volume
and increased subglottal air pressure.     Research suggests that glottal
resistance is the primary factor to  control low pitch,  while at higher
pitch levels, expiratory effort is more important.

Understanding of respiratory activity for  speech production has utilized an  important respiratory measurement called RELAXATION PRESSURE.
Relaxation pressure is the relationship  between subglottic air pressure
and lung  volume determined  when all  respiratory muscles  are relaxed.
The subglottic pressure results from the  recoil of the respiratory system that is created by tissue elasticity, surface tensions, and gravity.
Relaxation pressure measurements are determined for both inspiratory and
expiratory pressure.  To illustrate this concept of relaxation pressure,
take as deep a breath as possible (inspiration).  Do not exhale (glottis
closed) but try to relax as much as possible while maintaining lung volume.  You should be aware of expiratory pressures acting on the respiratory system.  Open the glottis and you exhale.   To understand the opposite relationship,  exhale  maximally and determine which  muscle forces
(inspiration or expiratory)  are at work.   Open the  glottis,  and you
inhale.

The plotting of this data in relationship to lung volume and subglottic air pressure  is referred to as the  PRESSURE-VOLUME DIAGRAM (Figure
25).    During sustained phonation  of a vowel,  there is  a point on the
graph  where relaxation pressure is  equal to  subglottic air  pressure
(where the  dashed line bisects the  solid line).   At  this theoretical
point no  muscular effort is  required to sustain  phonation.   However,
above or  below this point expiratory  or inspiratory muscle  forces are
necessary  to offset  either the  expiratory  or inspiratory  relaxation
pressures.

Gravity influences the  function of the respiratory  system.   From a
clinical standpoint, it is important to understand that relaxation pressure is  affected by body  position.  For  example,  the person  who is
standing or sitting  erect has the gravitational pull  inferiorly on the
chest wall and diaphragm.   In this  case expiratory pressure is exerted
upon the chest and inspiratory effect  is exerted on the diaphragm.   In
the supine  position the  pressure on  the chest  and diaphragm  undergo
expiratory influences.

The importance  of this  information to  the begining  student is  to
understand that  muscle activity  must constantly  change,  to  check or

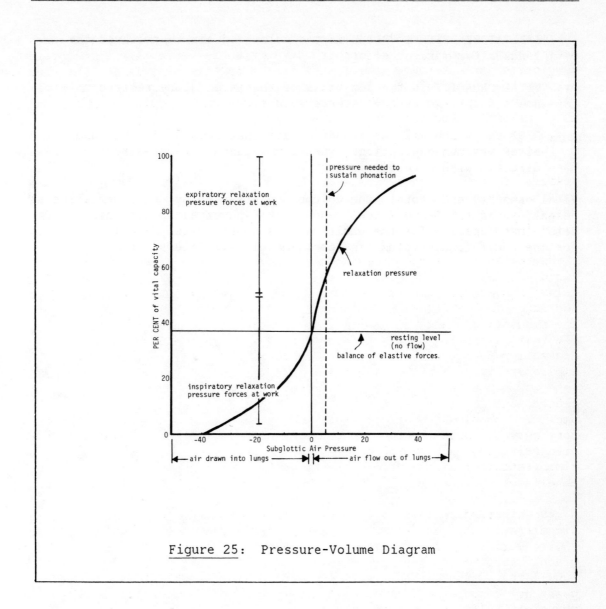

Figure 25:   Pressure-Volume Diagram

enhance elastic recoil forces,  in order to maintain constant subglottic pressure at  different lung volumes.  Failure  to do so will  result in unwanted fluctuations in loudness and pitch during speech.

Changes in  lung volume may be  measured with a  respirometer (Figure 26).  The volume  measures provide convenience in  describing pulmonary function.

- TIDAL VOLUME is the amount of air that enters and leaves the lungs during vegetation breathing.

- INSPIRATORY RESERVE VOLUME is the volume of air taken into the lung with maximum effort.

- EXPIRATORY RESERVE VOLUME is the volume of air that leaves the lungs after maximum effort.

- VITAL CAPACITY is the sum total of the inspiratory reserve volume and the expiratory reserve volume.

- RESIDUAL VOLUME is the amount of air that remains in the lungs after maximum expiration.  The volume can not be measured directly with a respirometer.

Vital capacity and  total lung volume are affected by  such variables as height,  weight,  temperature,  and general physical conditioning.   The total lung capacity for the adult male is approximately 6.0 liters,  and for the adult female volume is approximately 4.2 liters.

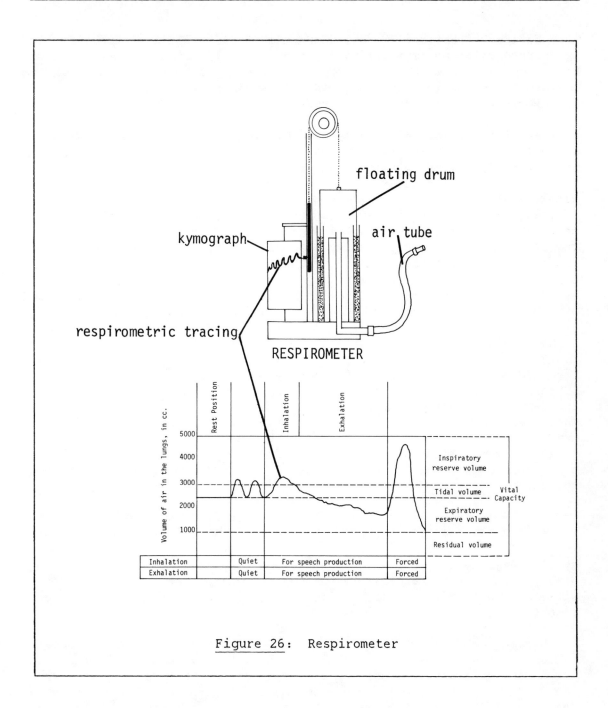

Figure 26:   Respirometer

## 2.4 Clinical Respiratory Conditions

There is a  developmental change in breathing patterns  during the first
year of life.   By about twelve months of age,  the child demonstrates a
prolonged expiration and quick inspiration  when phonating that is characteristic of adult speech breathing.   This is in marked contrast to the
rapid inspiration and expiration that  characterizes the newborn infant.

For both cry respiration and noncrying vocalizations, there is an apparent developmental increase in thoracic wall movement. Vegetative breathing is predominantly abdominal movement. Such respiratory changes for phonation during the first year are probably related to general motoric advances that accompany trunk and limb development.

Most of the time, very little thought is given to breathing. We simply do it. If, however, you have experienced swallowing too large a bite of food, or trying to talk while swallowing, you immediately realized the effects of not being able to breathe easily.

When we move from quiet vegetative breathing to controlled prolonged respiration for speech, a complex physiological network goes into operation. Respiration for speech requires coordination of anatomical structures that are controlled by the brain. Speech-language pathologists are often confronted with clients, such as the cerebral palsied, who have difficulty controlling respiration for speech. In fact, 40 to 80 percent of cerebral palsied individuals have breathing problems.

Most times, when the neuromotor system is not intact, there is a delayed response to voluntary efforts for speech. Speech can be affected because areas of the nervous system are damaged, creating disintegration of the neural signal for breathing. Also, respiration is influenced indirectly, by motor involvement of the tongue, vocal folds that create airway obstruction, or by lessened activity of the abdominal muscles and diaphragm. The results of these conditions may be slow and irregular expiration. Speaking, then, is characterized by reduced loudness or abrupt uncontrolled loudness, or by irregular and arrhythmic speech.

To aid individuals who have breathing difficulty, attempting to increase vital capacity serves little value. Speech is produced in the range of 10 to 20 percent of vital capacity. The total amount of air available is less important than efficient use of the existing air supply. Therapy is concerned with the controlled initiation and use of the airstream, with minimal air wastage, accomplished by the least physical effort.

Therapeutic techniques to facilitate respiration often use the body's reflex centers. Inspiration can be stimulated by temporarily impeding the client's airway. This is done by pinching the nostrils while the mouth is shut, or having the person hold his/her breath for as long as possible. Each maneuver creates an oxygen deficit that will trigger an inspiratory reflex. Other techniques include moving the arms and legs of the client. The intake of air in this manner may be essential for vocalization.

Seen in infants, reflexive vocalizations associated with expiration often accompany gross motor activities such as pulling, pushing, or eating. When a condition exists which effects the normal controlled expiration for meaningful speech, therapy may require the use of these activities as well,  aiding the  individual to  assume an  appropriate speech posture.   To adapt the client to the most advantageous body posture for speech, the therapist must understand and apply knowledge about the dynamic functions of all the muscles of respiration.

## Glossary

aerophagia:    Spasmodic swallowing of air, followed by belching.

alveolar:    Capillary membrane.

apnea:    Temporary absence of breathing.

aspirate:    Act of sucking in or sucking up.

Biot's Respiration:    Rapid, short breathing, with pauses of several
    seconds.

Cheyne-Stokes Respiration:    breathing characterized by rhythmic waxing
    and waning of respiration depth, with regularly recurring apneic
    periods.

dysapnea:    labored, distressful breathing.

expiration:    Breathing out; to exhale air from lungs.

Hering-Breuer Reflex:    Progressive stretching of alveoli cells; inhib-
    its inspiration, and brings about expiration.

pneumograph:    Any graphic display of respiratory movements.

pneumotachograph:    An instrument used to rcord the pressure or veloc-
    ity of air flow.

spirometer:    Any instrument used to measure the air capacity of the
    lungs.

tracheotomy:    The formation of an aritficial opening in the trachea.

U. R. I.:    Upper respiratory infection.

# References

Comroe, J. H., Jr., Forster, R. E., Dubois, A. B., Briscoe, W. A., & Carlson, E. (1962). The lung: Clinical physiology and pulmonary function tests (2nd ed.). Chicago: Year Book Medical.

Draper, M., Ladefoged, P., & Whitteridge, D. (1959). Respiratory muscles in speech breathing. Journal of Speech Hearing Research, 2, 16-27.

Hixon, T. J., Mead, J., & Goldman, M. D. (1976). Dynamics of the chest wall during speech production: Function of the thorax, rib cage, diaphragm, and abdomen. Journal of Speech Hearing Research, 19, 297-356.

McMinn, R. O. M. H., & Hutchings, R. T. (1977). Color atlas of human anatomy. Chicago: Year Book Medical.

Mysak, E. D. (1980). Neurospeech therapy for the cerebral palsied (3rd ed.). New York: Teacher's College of Columbia University.

Selkurt, E. E. (1982). Respiration. In E. E. Selkurt (Ed.), Basic physiology for the health sciences (2nd ed.). Boston: Little, Brown.

Sinclair, J. D. (1978). Exercise in pulmonary disease. In J. V. Basmajian (Ed.), Therapeutic exercise (3rd ed.). Baltimore: Williams & Wilkins.

Wiebel, E. R. & Gomez, D. M. (1962). Architecture of the human lung. Science, 137, 577-585.

Zemlin, W. R. (1968). Speech and hearing science, anatomy, and physiology. Englewood Cliffs, NJ: Prentice Hall.

# Chapter 3
# Larynx and Phonation

The larynx is the superior continuation of the respiratory passage.  The cartilaginous system is held together by membranes,  and within the laryngeal cavity  lie the vocal folds.   Muscles acting directly  or indirectly on  the vocal folds and  the cartilages of the  larynx,  together with air from the lungs, produce voice.  When sound is modified by other regions above the  larynx,  a quality of PHONATION results  that is distinctive to  each of  us.   When conditions  arise which  interfere with vocal fold and cavity vibration  (resonation),  voice quality may change to such a extent that the  voice calls attention to itself,  interfering with the communication process.

## 3.1 Skeletal Structure of the Larynx

The larynx is composed of nine cartilages and one bone (Figure 27).

1.  The HYOID bone can also be  considered as support for the tongue, as well as part of the laryngeal system.

    a.  It serves as an attachment for  many of the extrinsic laryngeal muscles.

    b.  The horseshoe-shaped hyoid is made of five parts:

    • Body (corpus).
    • Two greater cornua (major horns).
    • Two lesser cornua (minor horns).

2.  The THYROID is the largest cartilage of the larynx.

    a.  It is composed of two laminae  joined together in front to form an angle.

    b.  From the ANGLE  OF THE THYROID,  the laminae  diverge to a posterior width of approximately 43 mm.

    c.  The posterior  border of  each lamina  extends upward  and downward to form SUPERIOR and INFERIOR cornua.

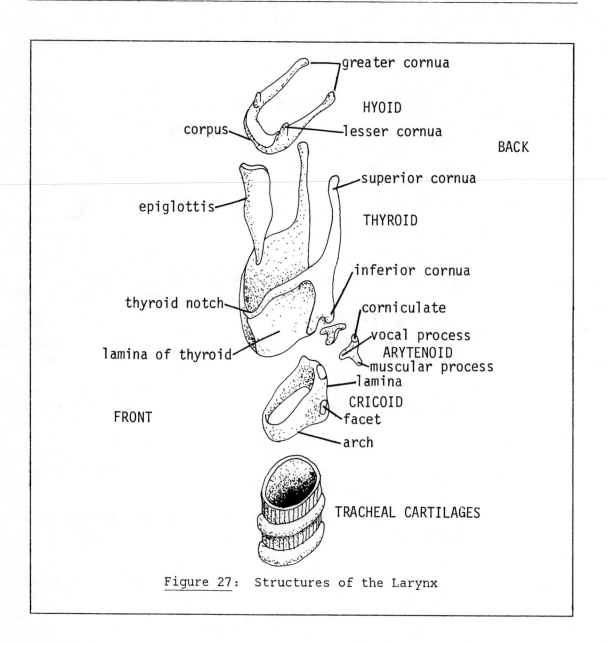

Figure 27:  Structures of the Larynx

    i.  Each superior cornua attaches indirectly to the corresponding major cornua of the hyoid.

   ii.  The inferior cornua attach to the posterior aspect of the CRICOID arch.

3.  The CRICOID cartilage is shaped like a signet ring with the anterior arch, a narrow convex ring, and posteriorly the lamina of "signet."

a.  The lamina extends  upward and lies between  the posterior aspect of the thyroid.

b.  The inferior  cornua of the  thyroid joins the  cricoid at articular facets near  the junction of the  lamina and the arch.

4.  Two ARYTENOID cartilages rest on the  superior border of the cricoid lamina.

a.  Each arytenoid approximates a pyramid in shape with

- A lateral projection is called the MUSCULAR PROCESS.
- An anterior projection is the VOCAL PROCESS.
- The superior aspect, or apex, curves slightly backward.

b.  The arytenoids  are capable of three  movements:   ROTARY, SLIDING, and TILTING.

5.  The  CORNICULATE cartilages  (cartilage  of  Santorini)  are  two pyramidal shaped  nodules located on  the apex of  each arytenoid for protection of the arytenoid.

6.  The CUNEIFORM cartilages (cartilage of  Wrisberg)  are rod shaped elastic cartilage found in the  posterior portions of the aryepiglottic folds to give support to that membrane.

7.  The EPIGLOTTIS is a single leaf-like structure bound by ligaments to the base of the tongue, walls of the pharynx, and thyroid cartilage.

a.  This structure acts to close off the laryngeal air way and deflect bulbus of food posteriorly into the esophagus during swallowing.

b.  In man's evolution it was, at one time, related to breathing by acting to seal the airway and prevent the intake of substance.

## 3.2 Laryngeal Membranes

1.  EXTRINSIC membranes  and ligaments  connect the  laryngeal cartilages, hyoid bone, and trachea (Figure 28).

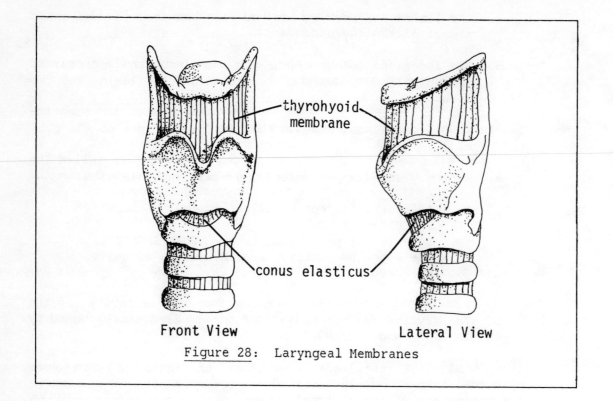

Figure 28:   Laryngeal Membranes

a.  Thyrohyoid membrane runs between the thyroid cartilage and hyoid bone.

    i.   The MIDDLE THYROID ligament  is the thickened anterior middle part of this membrane.

    ii.  The LATERAL THYROHYOID ligament is a thickened dorsal edge of the membrane.

b.  The HYOEPIGLOTTIC membrane runs from the epiglottis to the hyoid.

c.  The CRICOTRACHIAL ligament connects the cricoid to the first tracheal ring.

2.  The INTRINSIC membrane  covers the median surface  of the larynx, connecting the laryngeal cartilages together.

a.  The QUADRANGULAR  membrane runs between the  arytenoid and epiglottic cartilages.

    i.   A thickened fold along the  superior border of this membrane is called the ARYEPIGLOTTIC fold.

   ii. The thickened medial border is called the
     VENTRICULAR ligament.

 b. The CONUS ELASTICUS membrane is also part of the intrinsic
   membrane of the larynx.

    i. The anterior-midline thickened area of the membrane
      is the cricothyroid ligament.

    ii. The lateral aspects of the membrane are called the
      cricothyroid membrane, and extend upward from the
      cricoid cartilage to the vocal ligament.

## 3.3 Laryngeal Cavity

The laryngeal cavity is the upward continuation of the cavity of the
trachea from the cricoid cartilage to the superior entrance bounded by
the GLOSSOEPIGLOTTIC folds (Figure 29).

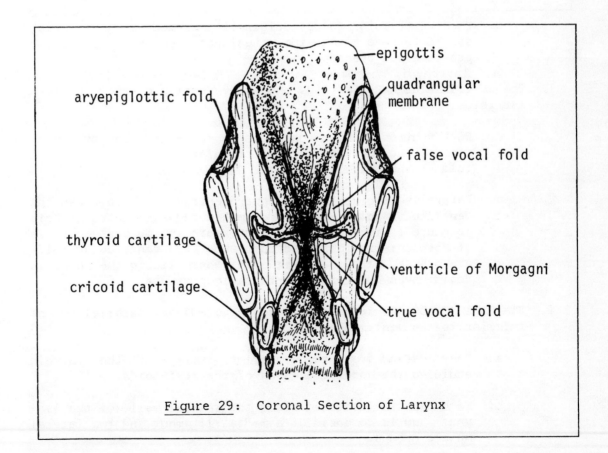

Figure 29: Coronal Section of Larynx

1.  The laryngeal cavity has three divisions.

    a.  The VESTIBULE, or superior subdivision, extends from the superior aperture of the larynx to the ventricular or false folds.

    b.  The middle subdivision, or VENTRICLE, extends from the ventricular folds to the true vocal folds.

    c.  The INFERIOR DIVISION extends from the vocal folds to the trachea.

2.  The larynx is a valving system. The VENTRICULAR FOLDS (paired) run horizontally along the lateral wall of the laryngeal cavity.

    a.  Each soft and somewhat flaccid fold contains the lower part of the quadralateral membrane with its ventricular ligament; mucous glands which, among other things, lubricate the vocal folds; and a few muscle fibers.

    b.  The ventricular folds are more widely separated than the vocal folds. That is, the opening between them is broader.

    c.  The ventricular folds originally formed a valve which served to keep air inside the lungs when excess intralung pressure was needed.

3.  The ventricle of MORGAGNI aids the valve action of the ventricular folds.

    a.  Each ventricle of Morgagni is a cave-like cavity having its opening between the ventricular fold and the vocal fold of that side.

    b.  Laterally it gives off an upward extension which, when the ventricular folds are approximated and the intrathoracic pressure is increased, the pressure inside the ventricle of Morgagni is increased and thus the ventricular folds are pressed harder against each other, aiding the folds to resist even greater intra-thoracic pressure.

4.  The VOCAL FOLDS, or true vocal cords (paired) are parallel to and inferior to the ventricular folds.

    a.  They extend from the posterior surface of the thyroid angle to the vocal processes of the arytenoids.

    b.  Each band is attached along the lateral wall of the larynx, and is composed of a medial ligament and two lateral muscle groups.

      i.  A VOCAL LIGAMENT and the upper part of the corresponding membraneous section of the conus elasticus.

     ii.  The THYROVOCALIS and THYROMUSCULARIS MUSCLES.

  c.  Its mucous membrane is thin and pale in color. Its median edge (vocal ligament) is pearly white.

  d.  The vocal folds form a valve which prevents the entrance of air or other substances into the trachea and lungs.

5.  The GLOTTIS (rima glottidis) is the opening between the vocal folds.

  a.  The intermembranous portion of the glottis is the anterior section bounded by the vocal folds.

  b.  The INTERCARTILAGINOUS portion is the posterior section bounded laterally by the medial surfaces of the arytenoid cartilages and posteriorly by the transverse arytenoid muscle.

  c.  The width of the glottis is determined by movements of the arytenoid cartilages.

      i.  When the arytenoids rotate so that their vocal processes are approximated, the glottis is narrowed.

     ii.  When the arytenoids slide toward each other the glottis is narrowed.

    iii.  The opening is widest during inhalation and narrowest during phonation.

  d.  Tilting the arytenoids, though it changes slightly the length of the glottis, is more important in affecting the tension of the vocal fold.

  e.  The length of the glottis may be altered by the rotating movements allowed by the crico-thyroid joint.

## 3.4 The Muscles of the Larynx

The laryngeal musculature is divided into two groups.

- EXTRINSIC muscles are those which support the larynx. They have at least one attachment on some structure outside the larynx.

• The INTRINSIC muscles control, among other things, phonation.
  They have both origin and insertion within the larynx.

The extrinsic muscles,  also called strap muscles,  function to move the
larynx as a whole (Figure 30).

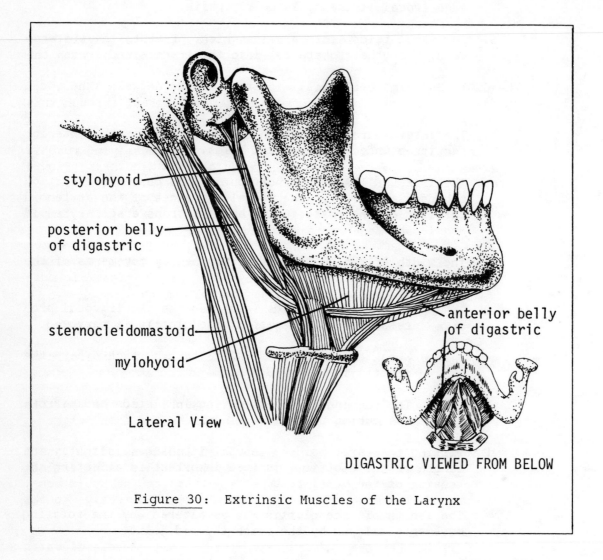

Figure 30:  Extrinsic Muscles of the Larynx

1.   Four muscles support the hyoid superiorly:

     a.   The DIGASTRIC is unique in that  it consists of two muscu-
          lar sections (bellies) joined by an intermediate tendon.

          i.   The ANTERIOR BELLY rises from the posterior surface
               of the mandible  near the symphysis and  runs down-

ward and inward to the intermediate tendon above the body of the hyoid.

    ii.   The POSTERIOR BELLY begins at the intermediate tendon, runs upward and to the mastoid process.

   iii.   The INTERMEDIATE tendon is fastened indirectly to the hyoid.

        1) A loop of tendon rises from the hyoid bone slightly anterior to its junction with the greater cornu.

        2) The intermediate tendon passes through this loop.

b.   The STYLOHYOID (paired) are slender muscles lying roughly parallel to the posterior belly of the digastric (Figure 30).

    i.   They originate at the styloid process of the temporal bone coursing downward and inward.

    ii.   Just above the hyoid, they split into two slips, which pass on opposite sides of the digastric muscle and insert on the body of the hyoid.

   iii.   The stylohyoid elevates and retracts the hyoid.

c.   The MYLOHYOID (unpaired) is a sheet of muscle fibers forming the floor of the mouth (Figure 30).

    i.   Its fibers rise along inner surface of the mandible and extend from the symphysis to the last molar.

    ii.   Its fibers course medialward and downward to insert into a tendinous MEDIAN RAPHE. This raphe extends from a point near the symphysis to the hyoid bone. The most posterior fibers attach directly to the body of the hyoids.

   iii.   When the mandible is fixed, this muscle elevates the hyoid bone and floor of the mouth in such acts as swallowing. It also holds the hyoid in position.

d.   The GENIOHYOID (paired), cylindrical muscles, lie on the superior surface of the mylohyoid (Figure 31).

    i.   The two geniohyoid muscles lie in contact with one another but on opposite sides of midline at the mandibular symphysis.

ii.   They diverge slightly as they run backward to insert on the anterior surface of the hyoid body.

iii.  When the mandible is fixed, the geniohyoids pull the hyoid forward and upward.

2.  Two muscle pairs support the hyoid bone inferiorly (Figure 32).

a.  The STERNOHYOID (paired) are flat muscles lying on the anterior surface of the neck.

i.   Each sternohyoid originates on the posterior surface of the manubrium sterni, and its fibers run upward to insert on the lower border of the hyoid body.

ii.  If the sternum is fixed, the sternohyoid draws the hyoid downward.

b.  The OMOHYOID are long, two-bellied muscles lying on the anterior and lateral surface of the neck (Figure 32).

i.   The SUPERIOR ANTERIOR BELLY begins along the lower border of the hyoid, runs downward and lateralward to an intermediate tendon.

ii.  The INFERIOR BELLY begins at the intermediate tendon which is held in position a little above the sternum and runs backward to the scapula.

iii. When acting from the scapula, it pulls the hyoid bone downward and somewhat backward.

3.  The THYROHYOID muscle supports the thyroid superiorly (Figure 33).

a.  It is a broad, thin muscle lying deep to the omohyoid.

b.  It originates at the oblique line on the thyroid lamina and runs upward to insert on the major horn of the hyoid bone.

c.  Contraction of this muscle lessens the distance between the thyroid cartilage and the hyoid bone.

4.  The STERNOTHYROID muscles (paired) support the thyroid inferiorly.

a.  They are long muscles that rise on the posterior surfaces of the manubrium sterni and the first costal cartilage, and run upward to insert at the oblique line of the thyroid lamina.

b.  Their function,  if the sternum is  fixed,  is to draw the
    thyroid downward.  They may also help to enlarge the phar-
    yngeal resonator by  pulling the larynx downward  and for-
    ward.

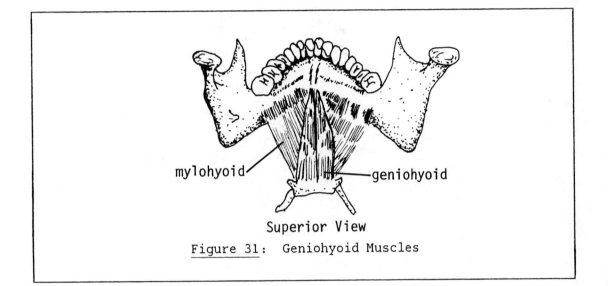

Superior View
Figure 31:  Geniohyoid Muscles

The INTRINSIC muscles may be divided according to function of opening or
closing the glottis (Figure 34).

1.  The abductor of the glottis  is the POSTERIOR CRICOARYTENOID mus-
    cle,  which is  situated on the posterior surface  of the cricoid
    cartilage.

    a.  It rises from a depression on the posterior surface of the
        cricoid lamina.

    b.  The fibers pass upward and  lateralward to converge before
        inserting on the posterior surface of the muscular process
        of the corresponding arytenoid.

    c.  It rotates  the artenoid so  that the muscular  process is
        drawn backward and the vocal  process outward.   The vocal
        folds thus are moved lateralward  and the glottis widened.
        The lateral fibers  of this muscle help  slide the aryten-
        oids lateralward.

2.  There are four adductor muscles which close the glottis.

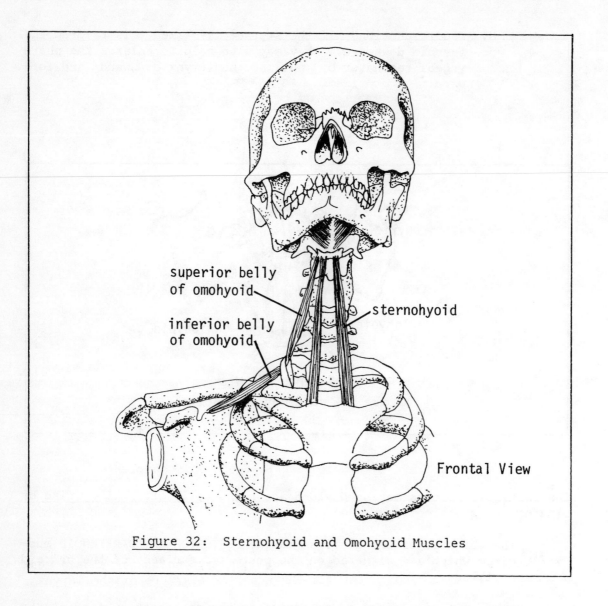

superior belly
of omohyoid

inferior belly
of omohyoid

sternohyoid

Frontal View

Figure 32:  Sternohyoid and Omohyoid Muscles

a.  The OBLIQUE ARYTENOID (paired)  originate on the posterior
    surface of the  muscular process of one  arytenoid (Figure
    35).

    i.  The fibers  run upward  and medialward,  cross the
        midline,  and  run to  the summit  of the  opposite
        arytenoid.

        1) Some of the fibers insert at this point.

        2) Others attach  to the  quadralateral membrane
           and to the lateral margin of the epiglottis.
           This  section  is  often  called  the
           ARYEPIGLOTTIC muscle.

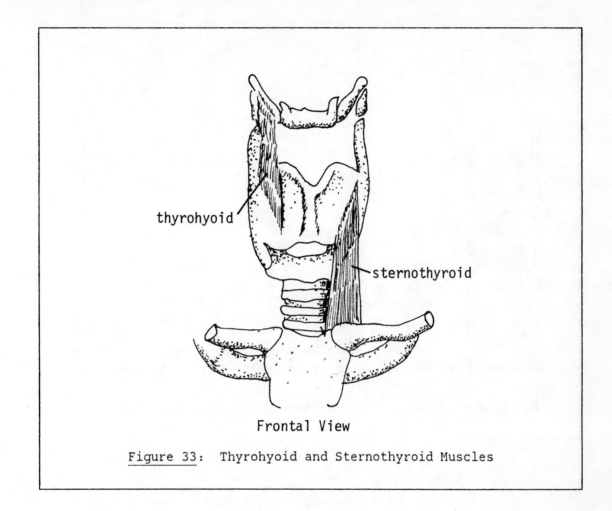

Frontal View

Figure 33:   Thyrohyoid and Sternothyroid Muscles

ii.   Together the two oblique arytenoids serve as a weak
sphincter for the superior aperture of the larynx.

b.   The TRANSVERSE arytenoid (unpaired) covers the entire posterior surfaces of the arytenoids, extending from the
bases almost to the summits (Figure 34).

i.   Its fibers rise along the muscular process and lateral edge of one arytenoid.

ii.   The fibers cross the midline and attach to the lateral border of the other arytenoid.   Some fibers
pass around the arytenoid and become continuous
with the thyroarytenoid muscle of that side.

iii.   The transverse arytenoid approximates the arytenoid
cartilages by sliding them toward one another.

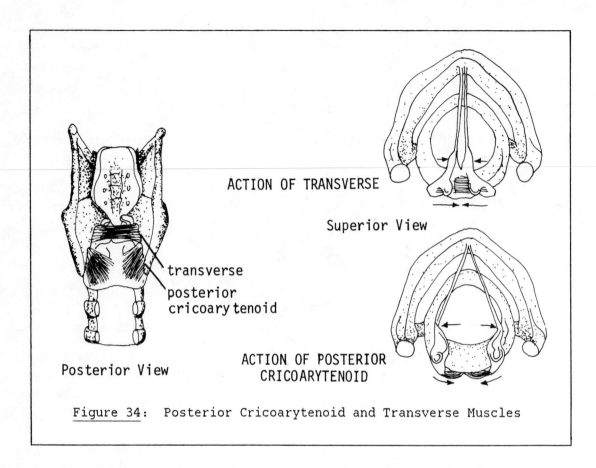

ACTION OF TRANSVERSE

Superior View

transverse

posterior
cricoarytenoid

Posterior View        ACTION OF POSTERIOR
                      CRICOARYTENOID

Figure 34:   Posterior Cricoarytenoid and Transverse Muscles

  1) This muscle closes the  posterior part of the
     glottis.

  2) For complete glottal closure it often must be
     helped  by the  lateral cricoarytenoid mus-
     cles.

c.  The LATERAL  CRICOARYTENOID (paired)  are located  deep to
the thyroid  cartilage in the  lateral wall of  the larynx
(Figure 36).

   i.  They rise from the upper borders of the arch of the
       cricoid and insert  on the anterior surface  of the
       muscular process of the corresponding arytenoid.

  ii.  They rotate the arytenoid so that the muscular pro-
       cess is drawn forward and the vocal process medial-
       ward.

d.  The  THYROARYTENOID (paired)   form the  substance of  the
vocal folds,  and include the thyrovocalis muscle and thy-
romuscularis fibers (Figure 37).

i.  They originate at the thyroid angle and insert from the vocal process  to the muscular process  of each arytenoid.

ii.  The action of these muscles  is to draw the arytenoid forward.  With the  oblique arytenoids, transverse arytenoid,  ventricular muscle,  and (possibly) the thyroepiglottic muscles, they complete the sphincter ring in the upper laryngeal wall.

iii.  They may  influence  the vibration  of  the  vocal folds.

1) By drawing the arytenoids  closer to the thyroid,    the  thyroarytenoids  make  the  folds more flaccid.

2) By varying the tension in  the walls to which the folds attach, the thyroarytenoids affect the mode of vibration of the folds.

3.  The CRICOTHYROID lies on the external surface of the larynx arising along the lower border and  outer surface of the cricoid arch (Figure 38).

a.  The muscle has two parts.

i.  The  anterior straight  part,  PARS RECTUS,  runs upward  to insert  along the  inner  aspect of  the lower margin of the thyroid lamina.

ii.  The posterior part, PARS OBLIQUE, angles upward and backward to  attach to  the inferior  cornu of  the thyroid.

b.  This muscle  increases the distance  between the  angle of the thyroid  and the arytenoids,   thus tensing  the vocal folds.  The PARS RECTUS may produce a rotation at the cricothyroid joint,  bringing the anterior  parts of the cricoid and thyroid cartilages closer together.

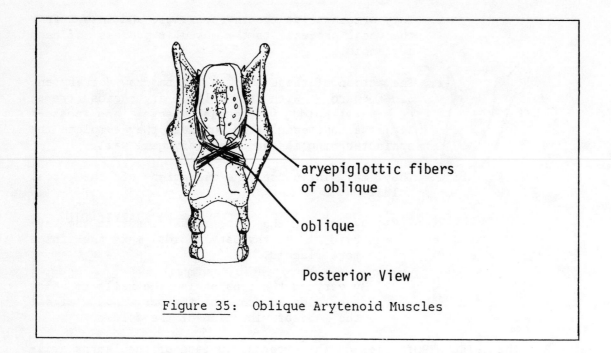

aryepiglottic fibers
of oblique

oblique

Posterior View

Figure 35:   Oblique Arytenoid Muscles

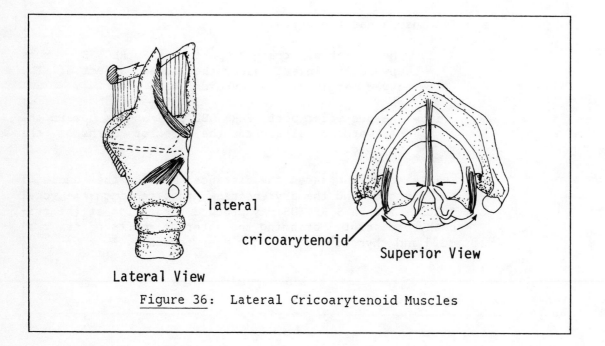

lateral

cricoarytenoid

Superior View

Lateral View

Figure 36:   Lateral Cricoarytenoid Muscles

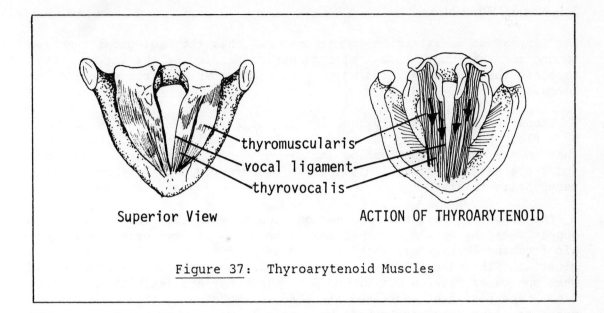

Superior View                    ACTION OF THYROARYTENOID

Figure 37:  Thyroarytenoid Muscles

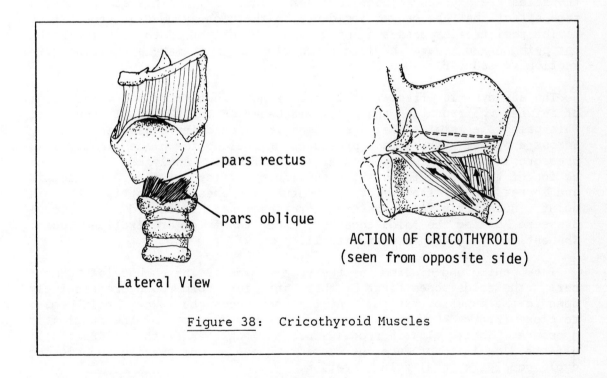

pars rectus

pars oblique

ACTION OF CRICOTHYROID
(seen from opposite side)

Lateral View

Figure 38:  Cricothyroid Muscles

## 3.5 Normal Phonation

The larynx, as an extension of the trachea, has the biological function to protect the lungs. The valving characteristics of the larynx serves to close the passageway and prevent foreign material from entering the lungs.

Phonation is a secondary function of the larynx. Voicing is produced by a flow of air through the glottis. By a dynamic set of circumstances that invoke muscle contraction and aerodynamic principles, the vocal folds are set in motion. This process is referred to as the myoelastic-aerodynamic theory.

The theory states that phonation occurs when the vocal folds are approximated by muscle contractions acting on the arytenoid cartilages. Air from the lungs increases in speed as it flows through the narrowed glottis. The same effect of increased air flow velocity is experienced when one walks between buildings on a windy day and feels the "rush" of wind. The result of increased air flow through the glottis is a drop in pressure along the margin of the vocal folds. When tissue pressure inherent within the folds exceeds the pressure at the glottal margin, the folds are "sucked" closer together (Figure 39). This action is the same effect that has caused accidents on the highway when a large, fast moving semi-trailer passes a small car. The driver of the car feels the car being drawn toward the larger vehicle and must make a steering correction to counter the pull.

The aerodynamic effect that is occurring, whether to the vocal folds or between the truck and the car, is based on the BERNOULLI principle. This principle states that as a gas or liquid increases in velocity across a plane, there is a pressure drop along the plane (i.e. less pressure is exerted perpendicular to the flow). Applying this to the action of the vocal folds, the continuing effect of narrowing glottis and increasing air flow velocity eventually closes the glottis. At this point, subglottic air pressure increases until it exceeds the tissue pressure holding the folds together, and the folds are exploded apart. The entire cycle then repeats itself.

The opening and closing of the vocal folds is in an undulating manner. The folds open first at their inferior border and progressively open to the superior margin. As the top opens the lower margin begins to close (Figure 40). As the folds are moved apart by the subglottic pressure, their elastic recoil forces, together with the Bernoulli effects, begin to produce the closing phase. One opening and closing cycle completes vocal fold vibration.

When describing the physical aspects of sound, the term frequency is used, however, when the perceptual aspect of sound is discussed the term pitch is used. Pitch, then, is directly affected by the frequency; the higher the frequency, the higher the pitch. There are three vocal registers within an individual's total pitch range. The range that is used

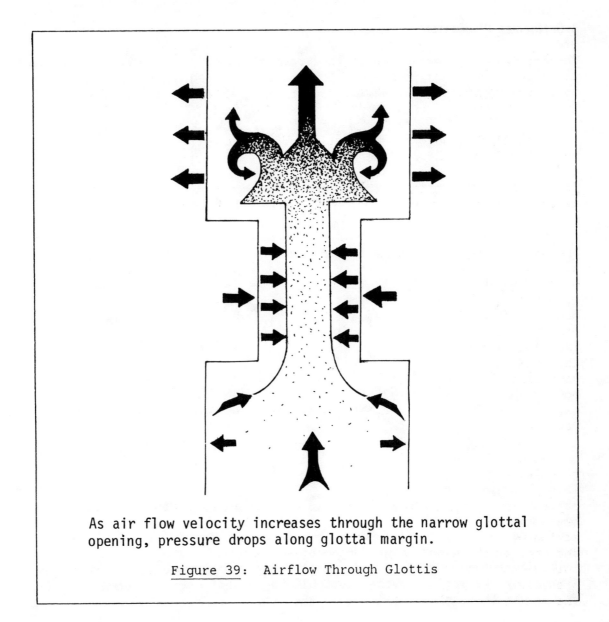

As air flow velocity increases through the narrow glottal opening, pressure drops along glottal margin.

Figure 39:  Airflow Through Glottis

for normal speech is referred to as the modal or chest range.  Falsetto, or head register, is the highest range.   The lowest range is called the VOCAL FRY, glottal fry, or pulse register.  Some individuals may produce vocal fry at the end of a sentence.   However, there is no apparent distinct physiological demarcation as  one  moves  from  one  register  to another, though a few individuals report feeling a laryngeal adjustment, particularly when going from the modal range to falsetto.

Pitch  changes  as  an  individual  becomes  older.    The  primary  area responsible for frequency changes lies with  the laryngeal area and specifically with  the vocal folds.   It has  been determined that  in the

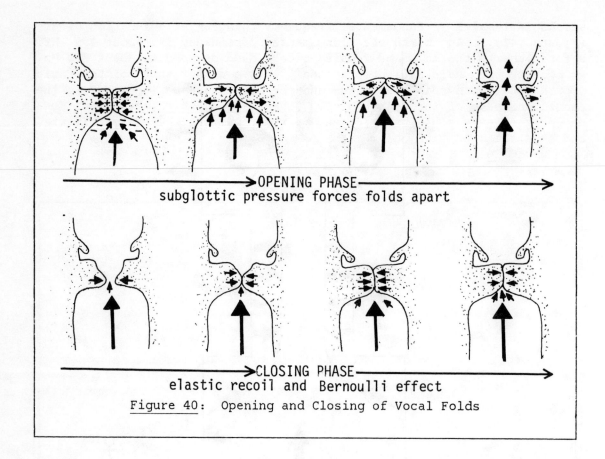

OPENING PHASE
subglottic pressure forces folds apart

CLOSING PHASE
elastic recoil and Bernoulli effect

Figure 40:  Opening and Closing of Vocal Folds

modal range, while laryngeal size is a determining factor in vocal pitch
and the length of the vocal folds contribute to fundamental frequency to
some extent,  the vibrating mass or thickness  of the vocal folds is the
greatest factor determining fundamental frequency.  The mass varies as a
function of the tension of the  vocal folds.  Presumably this is accomplished by the action of the  lateral and posterior cricoarytenoid,  and
by the lengthening of the folds by the cricothyroid.

Vocal fold vibration varies with pitch and loudness.  This is due, in
part,  to the unique anatomical makeup of  the folds.  Each fold can be
considered having  an outer covering and  medial edge whose  membrane is
less elastic than the body of the fold.  At low pitch there is a difference in the vibratory phase of these two tissue layers.  The difference
in motion can  be observed both in a lateral  and longitudinal direction
along each  vocal fold  when viewed from  above,  and  in a  superior to
inferior direction  when viewed  from a frontal  section.  As  pitch is
increased both layers increase tension,  mass of the folds is decreased,
and they begin to vibrate in synchronization.

The fundamental frequency of vocal fold vibration,  in the adult,  is
approximately 105-135  times per second in  males and 200-230  times per

second in females.   Fundamental frequency changes  as a function of age
(Figure  41).   At  birth  the  fundamental  frequency  is  about  400  Hz.
Before puberty the male and female voices  have dropped to about 280 Hz.
At puberty the  male will drop another  octave as a result  of the rapid
growth of  the thyroid  cartilage and the  simultaneous increase  in the
length and mass of the vocal folds.  Other factors which may effect fundamental frequency of the voice may be race, culture, heredity, climate,
and physical conditioning.

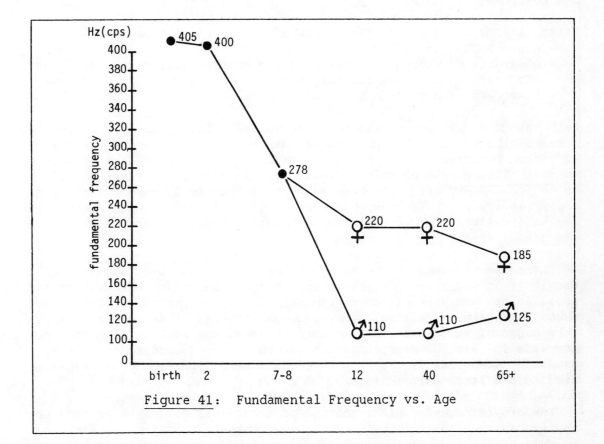

Figure 41:  Fundamental Frequency vs. Age

Fundamental frequency differences  are inherent in phonetic  units of
speech.   High vowels have a higher  fundamental frequency than low vowels.   This difference is explained by the combined effect of the larynx
and articulators on the vocal folds.  Vocal fold function is, therefore,
dependent on  phonemic utterance.   The  approximation of the  folds may
depend on the influence of abutting sounds.

Intensity changes constantly during  conversational speech.   Persons
give greater emphasis to certain syllables, words, or phrases.   To give
stress, intensity,  for example,  is increased by added subglottic pres-

sure (other factors that contribute to stress are DURATION and
FREQUENCY). However, subglottic air presure increases during conversation are not due to increased respiratory effort, but rather, to the
effects of the glottic opening and closing and laryngeal changes in the
supraglottal areas. It has been demonstrated that the same mechanical
maneuvers that increase subglottic pressure contribute to the distinction between consonant cognates such as /t/ and /d/.

## 3.6 Disorders of Voice

Voice disorders can be generally grouped into three categories:

- Disorders of increased vocal fold and/or laryngeal mass.
- Disorders of neurological origins.
- Disorders of psychosocial origins.

Each category is not necessarily exclusive. There may be a dynamic
interrelationship. The psychogenic disorder may produce a change in
laryngeal function which, in turn, results in changes in the structure
(mass). The reverse of this process may also occur. Further a child's
voice problem may actually begin as a true organic disease, such as an
upper respiratory infection, but because of prolonged illness, the child
may habitually learn to use a deviant voice, even after the infection
has disappeared.

Increased size and change of shape of the laryngeal mechanism, as a
result of an increase in tissue mass, changes the normal movement of the
vocal folds, and prevents them from properly approximating. Such vocal
abuse as excessive yelling, coughing, and throat clearing are the primary cause of voice disorders in both children and adults. An abnormal
increase in mass, however, may also be due to such conditions as laryngeal web, stenosis, virus, tumor, endocrine disorders, or a traumatic
blow to the laryngeal mechanism.

Inapproprate neurological control of the vocal folds and/or the laryngeal cavity results in voice disorders. These conditions, also known
as dysarthria, have distinctive vocal quality and motor characteristics.
Dysphonia may be one of the first signs of neurological voice problems .
A few common neurological conditions, of which deviant vocal productions
is apparent, include:

- Parkinson's Disease (can result in a hypokinetic dysarthria).
- Ataxia (caused by a lesion to the cerebellum of the brain).
- Apraxia of Phonation (results from a lesion in the expressive
  language area -- Broca's Area -- in the dominant cerebral hemi-
  sphere of the brain).
- Spastic Pseudobulbar Dysphonia.
- Flaccid Dysarthria (results in paralysis or weakness of the
  speech musculature).

Emotional and situational stress may cause abusive vocal behavior, which can result in an organic pathology of the laryngeal mechanism; or may result in a vocal quality which deviates from the norm to such an extent that it interferes with the communicative process. This sudden onset of deviant voicing may be due to externally or internally stimulated stressful situations. Terms used to describe these conditions are:

- Conversion aphonia.
- Spastic dysphonia.
- Immature personality.

Usually and uniquely, these voice deviations result without evidence of structural changes. A laryngeal examination would be normal. However, vocal nodules, ulceration of the vocal fold, or general edema of the laryngeal area may result.

## 3.7 Clinical Conditions

A person is considered to have a voice problem if his/her voice is characterized by disturbances of vocal quality, loudness, or pitch; or interference with the communicative process. Each of these attributes may be determined in part by the subjective assessment of the listener. The most common terms used to describe voice quality are "hoarseness" or "harshness". These terms can be misleading, and are probably best reflective of breathiness, pitch breaks, and restricted pitch range. Incidence studies suggest that hoarseness may be the most common voice disorder. Six to nine percent of school-age children have hoarse voices. Hoarseness lasting longer than two to three weeks should be viewed cautiously, and may require medical attention and voice therapy.

Hoarseness can occur as a result of vocal abuse and misuse, resulting in such pathologies as vocal nodules, polyps, vocal fold thickening, and generalized nonspecific edema. Common types of vocal abuse and misuse include:

- Shouting, screaming, and cheering, as experienced during play or sport activities.
- Strained vocalizations, such as excessive talking at loud or incorrect pitch levels.
- Coughing and throat clearing.

The degree of hoarseness perceived is related to the extent of the vocal abuse or misuse, and to the size of the existing pathology. Initially, edema of the outer margin of the vocal folds is caused by abusive undulating action of the vocal folds, and adds weight and stiffness causing transient vibrations. Continued abuse may result in this swelling being replaced by fibrous tissue, so as to form a vocal nodule, adding more mass, thus more transient vibrations which are perceptually heard as hoarseness.

Contact ulcers which may appear on one or both vocal folds near the posterior margin were at times considered to be almost exclusively caused by vocal abuse, or by males using too low a habitual pitch level. Ulcerations of the vocal folds may, however, be due to irritation of the fold mucosa from endotracheal tubes inserted during surgery; or, in the older population, from gastric fluids which may be regurgitated during sleep when the individual lies in the supine position.

Treatment of vocal fold pathologies which result from vocal abuse may require both medical intervention and vocal retraining by a speech-language pathologist. Surgical removal of vocal nodules, for example, without voice therapy, may result in the reappearance of the pathology because the abusive vocal behavior has not been eliminated. Often, vocal nodules may disappear with vocal rest and therapy without surgery when they are diagnosed early in their development.

Voice disorders characteristic of neurological problems often reflect the motor disability associated with the disease or lesion to the nervous system. Dysarthria is a term used to classify disorders of speech due to impairment of the nervous system which directly controls the muscles of speech.

## Hypokinetic Dysarthria

Hypokinetic dysarthria is most often associated as a symptom of Parkinson's Disease. It manifests itself in speech as monopitch, monoloudness, reduced stress, imprecise consonant production, short rushes of speech, inappropriate silences, variable rate, and harsh and breathy voice quality.

Early treatment with specific drugs may improve speech, as well as other symptoms. Traditional therapy concentrating on articulation, rate, and loudness may be a benefit, but realistic goals need to be discussed with the client. As the disease progresses (worsens), the role of the speech pathologist may be as a counselor rather than a therapist. Maintenance and, if needed, alternative means of communication, may be the most realistic therapy goals.

## Ataxia

Ataxia is caused by a lesion to the cerebellum of the brain that may occur before, during, or after birth. It can be characterized by postural disability, and a staggering gait; the movements are unsteady, and poorly coordinated. The ataxic patient produces speech that is uncoordinated, slurred, and lacking in rhythm. Perceptual deficits are also seen with ataxia, expecially with children, due to poor orientation of the body in space.

## Apraxia of Phonation

Apraxia of Phonation may result from a lesion in the region of the expressive language motor area (Broca's Area) in the dominant cerebral hemisphere. It is characterized by an inability to initiate volitional phonation at the laryngeal level. The patient may produce an unphonated airstream, with or without articulatory movements, or may produce articulatory movements without an airstream. The patient may only be able to exhale for vital purposes. Apraxia of speech (including phonation) may be a type of limb-kinetic apraxia, where the patient has lost the memory for the kinesthetic procedure needed for vocal tract functioning and the production of speech sounds. Apraxia of phonation appears as if respiratory and laryngeal movements can not be coordinated when an individual attempts to talk.

Treating apraxia of phonation may progress from throat clearing or coughing, to humming, to sustaining isolated vowel sounds.

## Spastic Pseudo-bulbar Dysphonia

Spastic pseudo-bulbar dysphonia results from a bilateral lesion of the upper motor neuron system. Such a lesion is associated with loss of discrete skilled movements, and with spasticity. Speech is characteristically hard, strained (due to overadduction of the vocal folds), of low monopitch, and reduced in intensity.

## Flaccid Dysarthria

Flaccid dysarthria is caused by a lower motor neuron lesion (spinal cord or below) which results in weakness, hypotonia, and muscle atrophy. As with most dysarthric conditions, therapy is focused on reducing rate of speech, over-articulating speech sounds, and varying pitch and loudness.

## Laryngectomy

Certain disease conditions or trauma result in amputation of the larynx. A laryngectomy is usually performed because of cancer. There are approximately 30,000 laryngectomees in the United States. These individuals breathe through an opening in the neck, called a stoma. Speech must be accomplished either by use of an electonic aid, or by using esophageal speech. Esophageal speech requires air to be taken into the esophagus, and forced back up like a burp. Sound is produced by the eructated air vibrating the structures of the oral cavity.

# Glossary

aditus laryngis:     That part of the laryngel cavity above the glottis.

aphonia:    Loss or absence of voice.

apraxia:    Loss of ability to execute voluntary acts.

bulbar paralysis:    Paralysis due to changes in motor centers of
     medulla; paralysis and atrophy of the lips, tongue, mouth, pharynx,
     and larynx muscles.

Cartilages of Santorini:    Another name given the corniculate carti-
     lages.

Cartilages of Wrisberg:    Another name given to the cuneiform carti-
     lages.

corditis nodesa:    Refers to "singers' nodules", or vocal nodules.

chorditis tuberosa:    A small whitish node on one or both vocal chords.

dysarthria:    A disorder of articulation due to impairment of the ner-
     vous system which directly controls the muscles of articulation.

dysphonia:    A general term referring to abnormal voicing.

esophagus:    The tube leading from the oral cavity to the stomach.

falsetto:    The highest voice register; also called the head register.

glottis:    The opening between the vocal bands.

glottal fry (pulsation):    The lowest register or voice produced by a
     syncopated beat of the vocal folds.

hyperkeratosis:   Growth or accumulated keratin (covering) formed on the vocal folds.

intensity:   The magnitude of sound, expressed in power or pressure.

laryngeal:   Relating to the larynx.

laryngitis:   inflammation of the larynx, usually resulting in hoarseness or loss of voice.

laryngology:   A study of the diseases of the throat, pharynx, larynx, nasopharynx, trachea, and the bronchial tree.

laryngoscope:   An apparatus used for visual examination of the vocal folds.

leukoplakia:   Growth often found on the vocal folds of smokers.

otolaryngology:   Specialty of medicine dealing with the ear and throat.

pitch:   The psychological perception of the frequency of a tone.

quality:   Refers to the complexity of the voice signal.

# References

Aronson, A. E. (1980).  Clinical voice disorders:  An interdisciplinary approach.  New York: Thieme-Stratton.

Boone, D. R. (1977).  The voice and voice therapy (2nd ed.).  Englewood Cliffs, NJ: Prentice Hall.

Bryce, D. P. (1974).  Differential diagnosis and treatment of hoarseness.  Springfield, IL: Thomas.

Darley, F. L., Aronson, A. E., & Brown, J. R. (1975).  Motor speech disorders.  Philadelphia: Saunders.

DeWeese, P. D., & Saunders, W. H. (1968).  Textbook of otolaryngology (3rd ed.).  St. Louis: Mosby.

Van Den Berg, J. (1958). Myo-elastic-aerodynamic theory of voice production.  Journal of Speech Hearing Research, 1, 227-244.

Wilson, D. K. (1972).  Voice problems of children.  Baltimore: Williams & Wilkins.

Wilson, F. B. (1972).  Voice disorders in children.  St. Louis: Jewish Hospital.

# Chapter 4
# Articulation — Structures of Resonation

Resonation refers to the vibration of a structure.  Articulation is the change of shape and position of structures to produce the sounds of speech.  Resonation is derived from the structures of articulation, that are inclusive of both the respiratory and the digestive systems.  Both structures are necessary for the production of vowels and consonants.

The pharynx is a structure of resonation and articulation.  Contraction of the pharyngeal muscles change the size and tension of the pharyngeal walls and change the vibrating (acoustical) characteristics of the system.  The mouth with its structures serves both resonating and articulation functions.  Changes in the oral cavity size and shape affect oral resonance.  The velum (soft palate) affects resonance by closing and opening the posterior port dividing the oral and nasal cavities.  In the English language the port is closed except for the production of /m/, /n/, and [ng] sounds, and vowels adjacent to these nasal consonants.  When conditions prevent the velopharyngeal port from adequately closing, hypernasal resonance may result.

## 4.1 Pharynx

1.  The PHARYNX is a wide canal about five inches long in the adult male that can be divided anatomically into three parts.

    a.  The NASO-PHARYNX is the most superior aspect located behind the nose.

    b.  The BUCCO-PHARYNX is the intermediate part behind the mouth.

    c.  The LARYNGO-PHARYNX extends downward behind the larynx, the most inferior muscle fibers reaching to the level of the cricoid cartilage.

2.  The pharynx consists of three overlapping pairs of constrictor muscles that are cased in an extensive aponeurosis (Figure 42). The posterior median aspect is known as the MEDIAN PHARYNGEAL RAPHE.

a. The INFERIOR CONSTRICTOR muscles are the strongest and largest of the constrictors.

    i. The most inferior fibers originate from the cricoid arch (these fibers are sometimes called the cricopharyngeal muscle) and the oblique line of the thyroid.

    ii. The fibers course backward and upward around the esophagus and meet their "opposite" from the other side at the median raphe.

b. The MIDDLE CONSTRICTOR is inferiorly overlapped by the inferior constrictor muscle and originates from three points: the greater cornua of the hyoid; the lesser cornua of the hyoid; and the stylohyoid ligament.

    i. The fibers course backward and upward to insert in the median raphe.

    ii. The superior fibers of the middle constrictor overlap the inferior fibers of the superior constrictor.

c. The SUPERIOR CONSTRICTOR muscles are regarded as the weakest of the constrictor muscles.

    i. Together with two facial muscles, the BUCCINATOR and OBICULARIS ORIS, they form a ring around the oral cavity.

    ii. The superior constrictor originates from two points: from the pterygoid plates of the SPHENOID bone; and from a ligament that runs from the pterygoid to the mandible called the PTERYGOMANDIBULAR RAPHE.

    iii. The most superior fibers insert into the velum.

d. The constrictor muscles function to move food downward in the esophagus.

e. For speech purposes, the constrictors act to increase tension on the throat region. Consequently, they change the vibration (resonation) of the supraglottic region.

f. Some individuals close the velophryngeal port by contraction of both the levator veli palatine and the superior fibers of the superior constrictor.

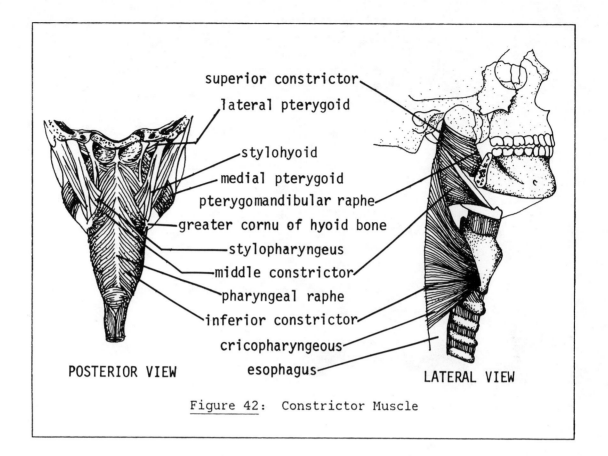

superior constrictor
lateral pterygoid
stylohyoid
medial pterygoid
pterygomandibular raphe
greater cornu of hyoid bone
stylopharyngeus
middle constrictor
pharyngeal raphe
inferior constrictor
cricopharyngeous
esophagus

POSTERIOR VIEW

LATERAL VIEW

Figure 42:  Constrictor Muscle

## 4.2 Palate

Palate Structure

The PALATE separates the oral and nasal cavities (Figure 43).

1.  The HARD PALATE is the bony "roof" of the mouth.

    a.  It is formed by the palatine  processes of the MAXILLA and
        by the horizontal aspect of the PALATINE bones.

    b.  The hard  palate is  covered by  a mucous  membrane tissue
        layer.

2.  The VELUM, or soft palate,  is the posterior muscular part of the
    palate.

    a.  It is attached  anteriorly to the posterior  margin of the
        hard palate and laterally to the walls of the pharynx.

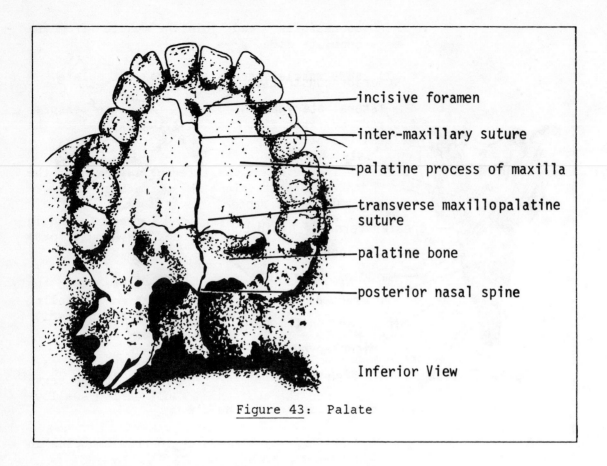

incisive foramen

inter-maxillary suture

palatine process of maxilla

transverse maxillopalatine
suture

palatine bone

posterior nasal spine

Inferior View

Figure 43:  Palate

b.  It extends posteriorly to a  conical projection called the
UVULA.

c.  The scaffolding of the velum  is the PALATINE APONEUROSIS,
to which several muscles attach.

d.  The muscles  of the velum act  to elevate and  retract the
structure to  close the  opening between  the naso-pharynx
and the oral-pharynx (Figure 44).

    i.  The LEVATOR VELI PALATINI, or soft palate elevator,
        (paired)  are  flat muscles  lying in  the superior
        lateral pharyngeal wall.

        1) They originate  at two  points:  the  petrous
           position of temporal bone;  and the cartila-
           ginous TORUS TUBARIUS  of the  eustachian
           tube.

        2) The fibers  run downward and  medialward into
           the velum, where they attach to the palatine

aponeurosis, and join the muscle from the opposite side.

3) These muscles act to lift the soft palate.

ii. The TENSOR VELI PALATINI, or soft palate tensors, (paired) are thin flat muscles lying lateral to the palatal elevator.

1) Their origin is the inferior surface of the sphenoid bone, along the eustachian tube.

2) The fibers run downward and forward to end in a tendon which loops around the hamular process.

3) The tendon then radiates medialward into the soft palate, where it attaches to its fellow of the opposite side and to the posterior margin of the palatine bone.

4) Upon contraction, they make the anterior part of the soft palate tense. They also serve to open the eustachian tube during swallowing.

iii. The GLOSSOPALATAL (paired) are narrow muscles in the GLOSSOPALATAL ARCH.

1) They rise from the posterior lateral margin of the tongue.

2) The fibers curve upward and radiate medially into the velum.

3) Upon contraction, these muscles either draw the soft palate downward, or raise the back of the tongue. Because of its point of insertion into the velum, it may have limited ability in elevating the tongue. The greatest mechanical advantage is to lower the velum.

iv. The PHARYNGOPALATAL (paired) are long muscles located in the PHARYNGOPALATAL ARCH.

1) Their origin is in the muscular wall of the laryngo-pharynx on the posterior margin of the thyroid lamina.

2) The fibers  run upward on the  medial surface
   of the pharyngeal musculature, and enter the
   velum.   Here they insert into the posterior
   margin of the hard palate,  the aponeurosis,
   and its fellow from the opposite side.

3) Some fibers  do not  radiate into  the velum,
   but rather continue to  a cartilaginous part
   of the eustachian tube.  This muscle portion
   is called the SALPINGOPHARYNGEAL.  Upon contraction it depresses the  soft palate.  The
   salpingopharyngeus portion serves to elevate
   the pharynx and dilates the eustachian tube.

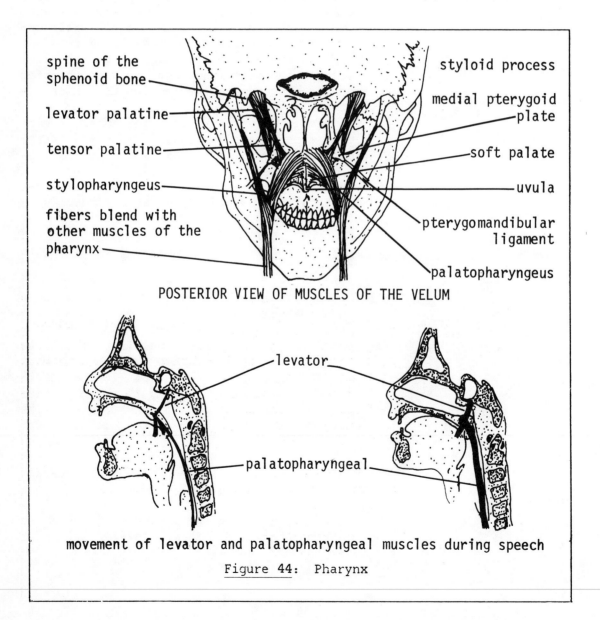

POSTERIOR VIEW OF MUSCLES OF THE VELUM

movement of levator and palatopharyngeal muscles during speech

Figure 44:  Pharynx

## Isthmus of Fauces

The ISTHMUS  OF FAUCES is  the passageway  connecting the mouth  and the pharynx.

1.  It is bounded above by the soft palate, below by the tongue,  and on the sides by PALATAL ARCHES (Figure 45).

2.  The GLOSSOPALATAL  ARCHES (also  called the  anterior pillars  of fauces)  are prominent folds of mucous membrane situated upon the inner surface of the lateral pharyngeal wall.  Each fold contains a glossopalatal muscle.

3.  Just posterior  to these  arches lie  the PHARYNGOPALATAL  ARCHES (called the  posterior pillars  of fauces).   They are  vertical folds of mucous membrane,  each containing a pharyngopalatal muscle.

4.  As the two muscles exit from the soft palate to the side walls of the pharynx  they separate,   forming a  depression in  which are situated the palatine tonsils.

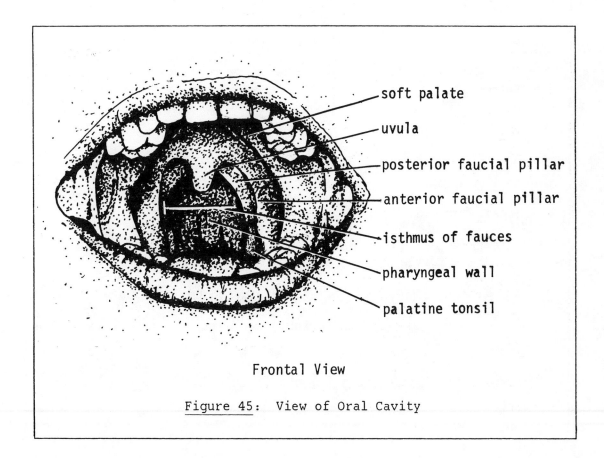

soft palate

uvula

posterior faucial pillar

anterior faucial pillar

isthmus of fauces

pharyngeal wall

palatine tonsil

Frontal View

Figure 45:  View of Oral Cavity

## 4.3 Tonsils

1.  The tonsils are a series of lymphoid tissue forming a circular band surrounding the openings into the oral pharynx.

    a.  The PALATINE TONSILS (paired) are oblong masses of variable size.

        i.  They lie in the space between the palatal arches.

        ii. Their medial (pharyngeal) surfaces, which are covered by mucous membrane, are exposed and present a number of orifices leading into crypts, or recesses, in the body of the tonsils.

    b.  The PHARYNGEAL TONSIL (unpaired), also called adenoid, is at the upper end of the pharynx, lying on its posterior wall.

        i.  It is a collection of lymph nodules over which the mucous membrane is thickened.

        ii. It is most distinct during childhood and becomes shriveled (or entirely disappears) in adult life.

    c.  The LINGUAL TONSIL (unpaired) is an aggregation of rounded lymph follicles covering the whole root of the tongue.

2.  The tonsillar ring serves a protective function by arresting infection.

## 4.4 Tongue

### Structure of the Tongue

The TONGUE (unpaired) is a mass of muscles covered by mucous membrane and containing a little fat and a few glands (Figure 46).

1.  Its form is roughly that of a boot turned upside down.

    a.  The tongue ends anteriorly in a flat, rounded tip called the APEX.

    b.  Posteriorly the apex blends without differentiation into the CORPUS or body of the tongue.

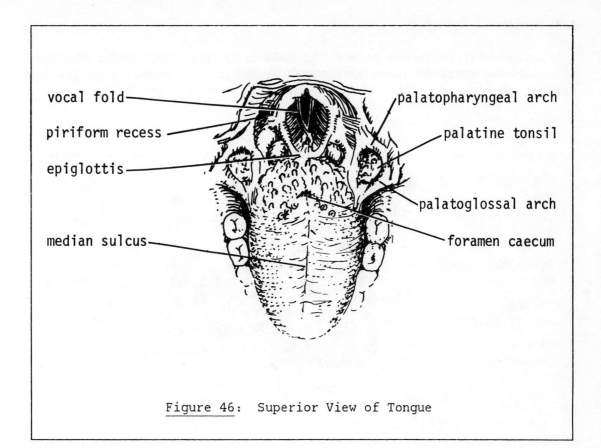

vocal fold

piriform recess

epiglottis

median sulcus

palatopharyngeal arch

palatine tonsil

palatoglossal arch

foramen caecum

Figure 46:   Superior View of Tongue

 

    i.   The upper surface of the  tongue is called the ORAL DORSUM.

   ii.   The sides of the tongue are the LATERAL MARGINS.

  iii.   Superfically the corpus is  separated from the ROOT of the tongue by the sulcus terminalis.

   iv.   Through the  root of  the tongue  pass the  muscles which connect it with the hyoid bone and the mandibular symphysis.

2.  The LINGUAL SEPTUM (unpaired)   divides the tongue longitudinally into two bilateral symmetrical parts.

    a.   The septum is narrow connective tissue lying in the median plane and surrounded on all sides by muscles.

    b.   It does not  quite reach the dorsum of  the tongue,  being separated from it by the superior longitudinal muscle.

Extrinsic Muscles of the Tongue

The muscles of the tongue are divided into EXTRINSIC and INTRINSIC groups. The extrinsic muscles have their origins outside the tongue and produce changes in SHAPE and POSITION of the tongue (Figure 47).

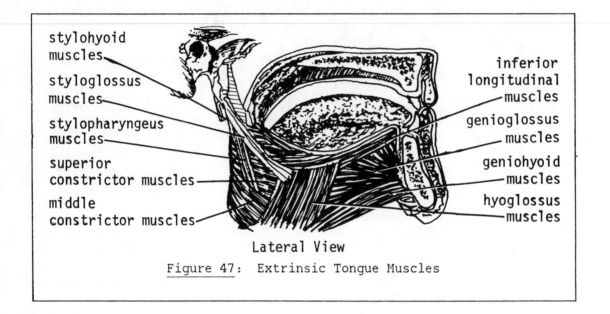

Lateral View

Figure 47: Extrinsic Tongue Muscles

1.  The GENIOGLOSSUS (paired) are fan-like muscles.

    a.  They rise from the posterior aspect of the symphysis of the mandible.

    b.  Their fibers insert into two primary regions.

        i.  The lowest fibers attach to the body of the hyoid.

        ii. Most of the fibers radiate to the dorsum of the tongue, where their insertion extends from tip to base.

    c.  Upon contraction, these muscles project the tip of the tongue forward and depress the whole organ in the floor of the mouth.

2.  The HYOGLOSSUS (paired) are quadralateral shaped muscles extending from the hyoid bone to the side of the tongue.

    a.  They originate along the major horn and body of the hyoid.

b. Their fibers run upward and slightly forward to the posterior part of the side of the tongue.

c. Here the hyoglossus turn and run forward between the inferior longitudinal and styloglossus muscles.

d. The hyoglossus draw the tongue backward and downward.

3. The STYLOGLOSSUS (paired) are elongated muscles extending from the styloid process to the apex of the tongue.

   a. They rise from the styloid process and stylohyoid ligament.

   b. They run downward, forward, and medialward to the hyoglossus, where they divide into two bundles.

      i. The larger, upper bundle turns to run longitudinally forward just below the lateral surface of the tongue, inserting within the mass of the tongue.

      ii. The smaller, lower bundle turns medialward, perforates the hyoglossus and ends in the posterior part of the tongue.

   c. These muscles function to elevate and retract the tongue.


Intrinsic Muscles of the Tongue

The INTRINSIC muscles, located entirely within the tongue, produce ONLY changes in SHAPE (Figure 48).

1. The SUPERIOR LONGITUDINAL muscle (unpaired) is a continuous layer of longitudinal fibers lying immediately beneath the mucous membrane, and occupying the entire dorsum of the tongue from tip to root.

   a. Its fibers are without definite origin or insertion.

   b. Upon contraction, it bulges the tongue upward in a longitudinal direction.

2. The INFERIOR LONGITUDINAL muscles (paired) run longitudinally through the inferior lateral part of the tongue.

   a. Their fibers originate at the mucous membrane of the root of the tongue. These fibers course forward, converging to form a bundle which runs toward the apex along with the styloglossus muscle.

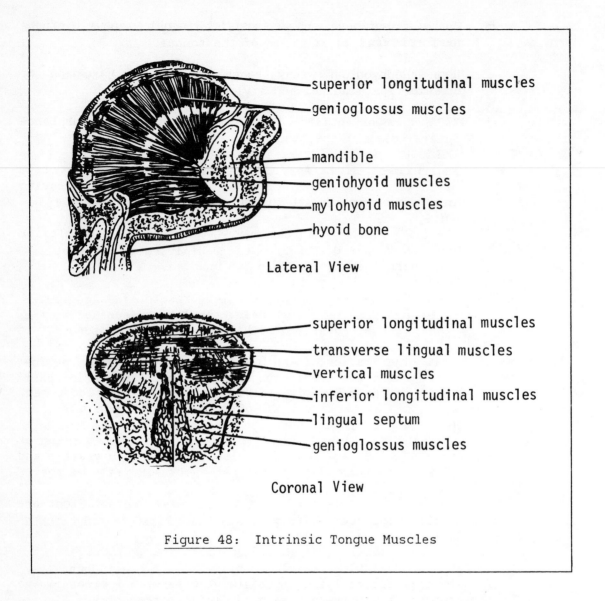

superior longitudinal muscles
genioglossus muscles

mandible
geniohyoid muscles
mylohyoid muscles
hyoid bone

Lateral View

superior longitudinal muscles
transverse lingual muscles
vertical muscles
inferior longitudinal muscles
lingual septum
genioglossus muscles

Coronal View

Figure 48:  Intrinsic Tongue Muscles

b.  Most of  the fibers  run straight  forward to  end in  the
    mucous membrane  of the  inferior lingual  surface.   Some
    bend upward to end in the mucous membrane of the dorsum.

c.  These muscles act to shorten the tongue.

3.  The TRANSVERSE muscles (paired) form the substance of the tongue.

a.  They consist of horizontal layers of fibers which run lat-
    eralward to the mucous membrane  of the  dorsum and lateral
    margins of the tongue.

b.  While some fibers  arise from the lingual  septum,  others perforate it.

c.  Upon  contraction,  they  narrow the  tongue,  bulging  it upward.

4.  The VERTICAL muscles (paired)   constitute the muscular substance of the lateral part of the tongue.

a.  Their fibers rise  from the mucous membrane  of the dorsum of the tongue and course downward and lateralward, weaving into the other lingual muscles.

b.  The fibers insert  in the mucous membrane  of the inferior aspect.

c.  The muscles flatten the tongue.


## 4.5 Teeth

The teeth are  arranged in two curved  rows on the upper  and lower jaw. The teeth appear in two successive sets, or dentitions (Figure 49).

1.  The twenty MILK, or BABY TEETH, erupt during infancy beginning at about six months  of age and continuing to about  two years;  and are shed during childhood, beginning at about six years of age.

2.  The thirty-two PERMANENT teeth replace the milk teeth.  Eight are found in each half of each jaw.

a.  The two medial, straight edged teeth are INCISORS.

b.  To the side of and a bit behind the lateral incisor is the strong, long somewhat pointed CANINE tooth.

c.  Behind  the canine  tooth  are  two PREMOLARS  with  broad uneven chewing surfaces.

d.  Behind the premolars are the three MOLAR teeth whose broad chewing surfaces carry four tubercles.

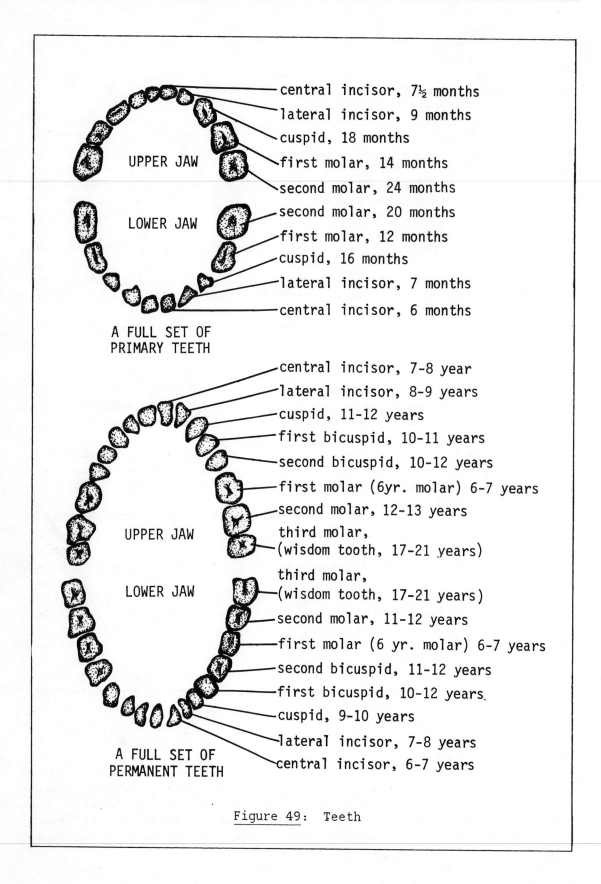

central incisor, 7½ months
lateral incisor, 9 months
cuspid, 18 months
first molar, 14 months
second molar, 24 months

UPPER JAW

second molar, 20 months
first molar, 12 months
cuspid, 16 months
lateral incisor, 7 months
central incisor, 6 months

LOWER JAW

A FULL SET OF
PRIMARY TEETH

central incisor, 7-8 year
lateral incisor, 8-9 years
cuspid, 11-12 years
first bicuspid, 10-11 years
second bicuspid, 10-12 years
first molar (6yr. molar) 6-7 years
second molar, 12-13 years
third molar,
(wisdom tooth, 17-21 years)

UPPER JAW

third molar,
(wisdom tooth, 17-21 years)
second molar, 11-12 years
first molar (6 yr. molar) 6-7 years
second bicuspid, 11-12 years
first bicuspid, 10-12 years
cuspid, 9-10 years
lateral incisor, 7-8 years
central incisor, 6-7 years

LOWER JAW

A FULL SET OF
PERMANENT TEETH

Figure 49:  Teeth

## 4.6 Physiological Implications -- Tongue and Velopharynx

From a physiological standpoint, the articulators are not separable independent speech structures. There is a dynamic relationship -- an interdependance -- that exists between each structure. Historically, phonetic theories were postulated on the relationship between one articulator (tongue) and a phonetic unit (vowels). The vowel triangle (Figure 50) has been used to demonstrate this relationship, and it has been inferred, if not espoused, that such production was uniform for all speakers of the English language. Data now indicate that tongue placement for vowels may vary from speaker to speaker, and within the same speaker. A factor such as lip position and degree of jaw opening will affect tongue position. Tongue position for a given vowel is influenced by the phonetic environment in which the vowel is placed and the rate of utterance. Of course, placement of the tongue affects the shape of the vocal tract and this may be the most significant factor in producing the identifiable vowel.

Some vowels are produced with longer duration than others and with the tongue achieving greater excursion to an extreme position. These are known as TENSE vowels. Vowels of shorter duration and produced with less extreme movements are called LAX vowels. Contrasting the vowels /i/ and /I/ is an example of tense and lax vowels.

A diphthong is a vowel with changing resonance. To produce diphthongs such as /eɪ/, as in play, or /aʊ/ as in how, requires a change in the vocal tract. The physiological changes required are often quite subtle and are more easily "heard" than "felt" during production.

The sounds /w/, /j/, /r/, and /l/ are semivowels that are resonant like vowels but are classified as consonants. Semivowels are subdivided into GLIDES (/j/ and /w/) and LIQUIDS (/l/ and /r/). In English, semivowels are used to release a vowel or diphthong ([rain], [yet]). In these examples, the semivowels precede the vowel to make a syllable and are characterized by a slight approximation of the articulators.

Consonants differ from vowels because the vocal tract is more constricted. Typically, they are produced with an aperiodic sound generated in the oral cavity. Tongue position may vary considerably to produce specific consonants. Production of the [s] may be made with the tongue tip elevated or lowered (Figure 51). Either position results in the production of an acceptable phoneme. The tongue is capable of changing position within the oral cavity, as well as assuming various shapes. The [r], for example, may be made with several tongue shapes but with a common position (area of constriction). It is readily recognizable as the intended sound because the tongue is being placed in a common position (Figure 52). Further, a portion of the tongue may be position-constant (e.g. dorsum or root) during repetition of a consonant

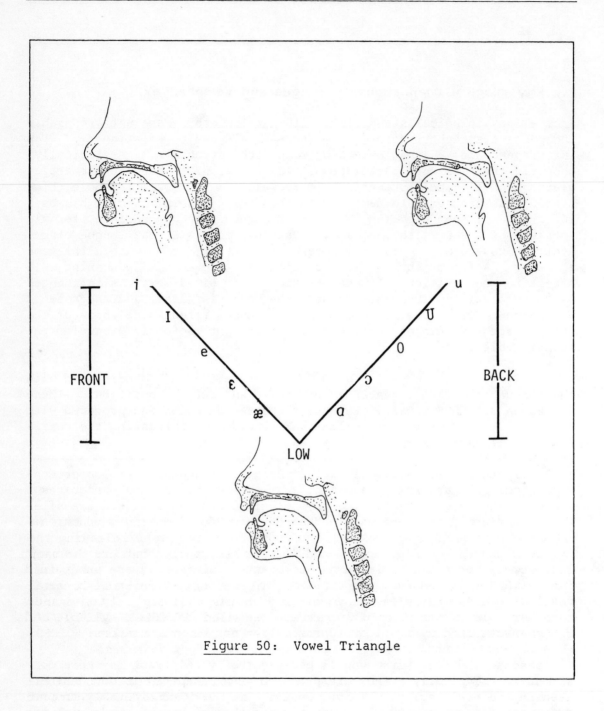

Figure 50:   Vowel Triangle

while another  aspect (tongue tip)  may  vary depending on  the phonetic
environment of  the consonant.    The tongue also  is influenced  by jaw
position.    The  degree of jaw opening  will affect where the  tongue is
positioned and how far the tongue must move.

Consonants are  classified into three  categories according  to their
manner of production:    stops (plosives),  fricatives,  and affricates.

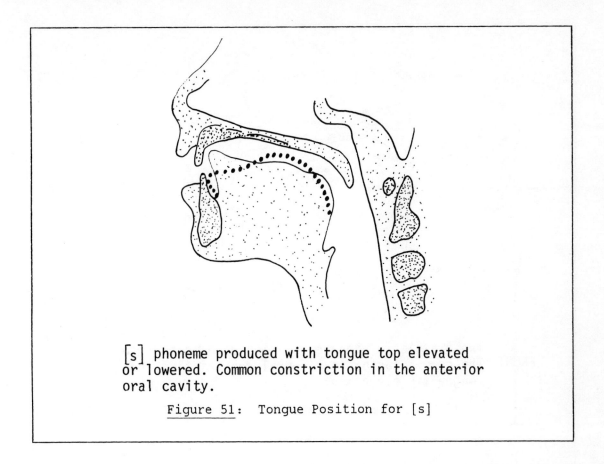

[s] phoneme produced with tongue top elevated or lowered. Common constriction in the anterior oral cavity.

Figure 51:   Tongue Position for [s]

Stop consonants are produced by a blocking of air flow with the lips or tongue, increasing air pressure in the oral cavity, then releasing the impounded breath with an explosive burst of air. In English the stop consonants are /p, b, t, d, k, g/, as in the words pie, by, tea, doe, crow, go. Half of the stop consonants listed are produced without vocal fold vibration (contrast the production of pie and buy). Consonants produced without vocal fold vibration are called VOICELESS (/p/, /t/, /k/); consonants produced with vocal fold vibration are called VOICED. All consonants can be categorized as either voiced or voiceless.

Technically, the relationship between vocal fold vibration and the opening of the vocal tract (stop-release) is the identifying feature of sounds voiced or voiceless. The timing of the stop release and the onset of voicing is known as VOICE ONSET TIME (Figure 53). Voiceless stops are acoustically distinguished from voiced stops by the delay in the onset of voicing and by the noise associated burst with release of the stop. Voiceless stops are produced with greater intravocal air pressure than voiced stops. Consequently, voiceless stops are released with a greater explosion of air.

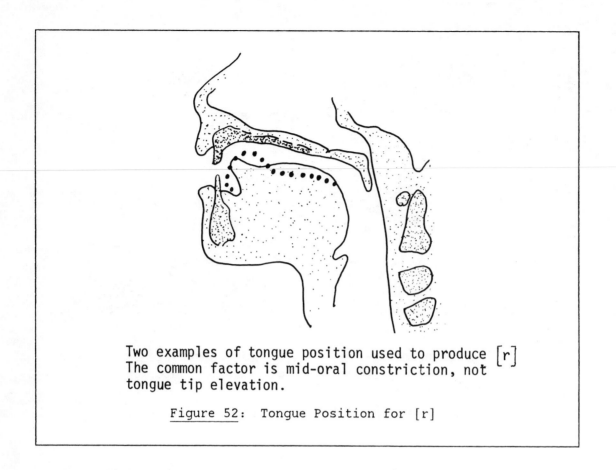

Two examples of tongue position used to produce [r]
The common factor is mid-oral constriction, not
tongue tip elevation.

Figure 52:  Tongue Position for [r]

Fricative consonants are acoustically characterized by the "friction" noise created by the compression of air flow through a narrow passage. Fricatives are produced and categorized by constriction created between the lips and teeth (labiodental), tongue and teeth (linguodental), tongue and gum ridge (palatal). Sounds classified as fricatives in English are /s/, /z/, /f/, /v/, /θ/, /ð/, /ʃ/, /ʒ/, and /h/. Fricatives are also voiced or voiceless. Unlike stops, however, these sounds can be prolonged and are also called CONTINUANTS.

Consonants that combine the production components of a stop with a fricative release are called AFFRICATES. There are two affricates in English, /tʃ/ and /dʒ/, as in the words "church" and "judge".

Another consonant category is nasal sounds. Nasals (/m/, /n/, /ŋ/) differ from other consonants because they are typically characterized by a periodic, vowel-like sound. These sounds are produced by the resonation of the entire vocal tract including the nasal cavity. The point of constriction for nasals is the oral cavity, which is blocked during production, while the velopharynx is open. All nasals are voiced in English.

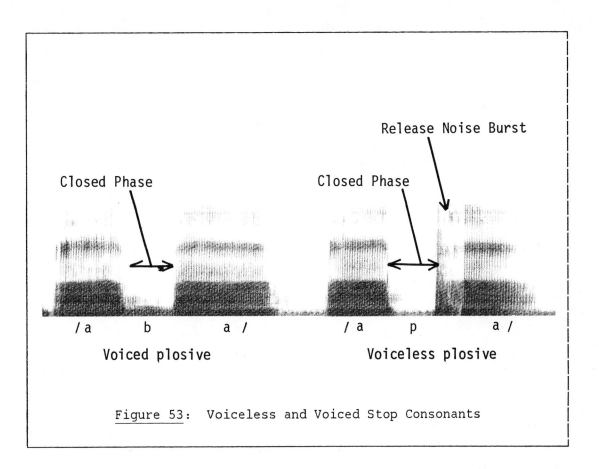

Figure 53:  Voiceless and Voiced Stop Consonants

The velum  and pharynx are articulators  that function in  concert to open or close the nasal cavity, from the oral cavity.  For normal speaking individuals the velum functions rather consistently.   The extent of velar movement and  speed of movement are influenced by  both tongue and lip movement.   For example,  the individual  who has little movement of the lips  and tongue during connected  speech (mumbler)  may  have relatively little  movement of the  velum.   This  will result in  a greater degree of nasal coupling than would be normally expected.

Velar excursion  also varies  according to  the phonetic  environment (Figure 54).    Greater velar  height is  achieved on  vowels with  high tongue carriage than with low tongue  position.   The velum also remains in a relatively low position when the vowel is in a nasal phone environment.  However, while velar height is fairly constant for the production of nonnasal consonants,  velar height increases during the production of nonnasal high pressure consonants, such as fricatives and affricates.

Velar  position is  determined by  the dynamic  relation between  the levator veli palatine, palatoglossus,  and the palatopharyngeus muscles, and the  tendency for the  mechanism to return  to its resting  state by elastic recoil.   The intensity of muscular  action may be determined by

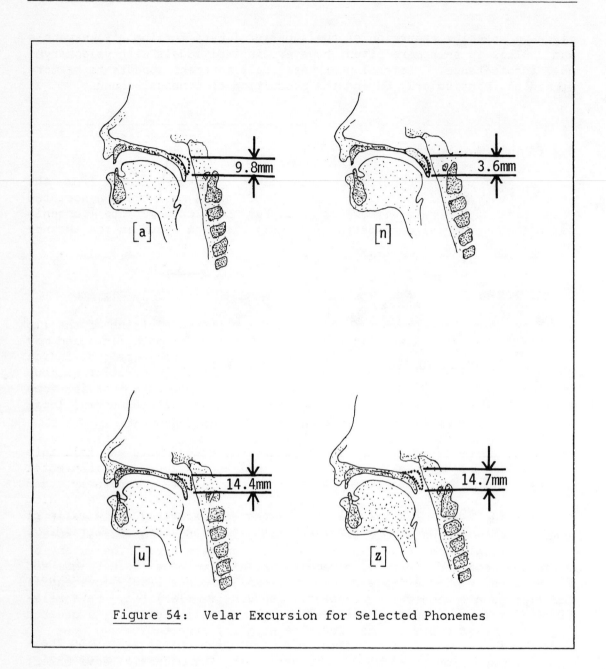

Figure 54:  Velar Excursion for Selected Phonemes

the position of the velum or tongue  position.   In either case,  it has
been suggested  that biomechanical control  of the  velum is due  to the
balance between muscular and nonmuscular  forces rather than simple muscular force producing directional movement.

The degree of  pharyngeal movement associated with  velar movement is
examined in  terms of posterior  pharyngeal wall and  lateral pharyngeal
wall excursion.   It is generally agreed  that in normal  speakers very
little posterior pharyngeal wall movement is evidenced.   A few speakers

may have anterior excursion of the superior fibers forming a Passavant's pad.   This is seen more often, however, in individuals with velopharyngeal incompetence.   Lateral pharyngeal wall movement appears to be more prominent, particularly during the production of nonnasal sounds.

## 4.7 Clinical Applications

The most common conditions that affect resonance result from the improper valving of the velum.   This condition is most often associated with cleft of the palate; however, velopharyngeal incompetence (congenital palatopharyngeal incompetency, or CPI) also can occur in the absence of clefting.

### Cleft Palate

Cleft palate is a term that is  generally applied to clefting of the lip and palate.  Cleft of the lip may involve one side or both sides and may or may  not involve the palate.   Because of the normal  palatal fusion process,  clefting of  the hard palate will generally  not occur without clefting of the velum.   When clefting of the velum occurs,  or for some reason the muscles of the soft palate fail to attach at the normal location, the velum cannot be elevated properly during speech.

The cause of cleft  palate is not fully understood but  may fall into such categories as mutant genes, chromosomal aberrations,  environmental teratogens  or inheritance.    It  affects  males more  frequently  than females and occurs at a frequency of one in 1000 births.   There is also evidence of racial  differences,  occurring approximately at  a ratio of 1:600 in Caucasians; 1:450 in Asians; and 1:2000 in American Negroid.

A subform of clefting is bufid uvula.  Bifid uvula refers to the congenital dividing of the uvula.  This condition occurs in about 1:72 normal speakers.   In some individuals, it may be an important indicator of possible velopharyngeal incompetence.

There are children with normal vocal  resonance prior to having their tonsils and adenoids removed,   who afterward demonstrate hypernasality. In such children the swollen adenoid mass may have masked velar incompetence, e.g., the velum could not obtain adequate closure but the swollen adenoid pad aided in completing the closure of the nasal port.  The professional,  noticing a bifid uvula in a  child who is to undergo removal of his/her tonsils, should be alert to potential velopharyngeal incompetency and perform more extensive evaluations.

Treatment  for   cleft  palate  and/or   velopharyngeal  incompetence requires the team effort of  professionals such as surgeons, dentists, and speech-language pathologists.  Surgery to close the cleft palate may not always result in sufficient velopharyngeal valving.  Basically, re-

mediation of the problem lies within  one or a combination  of treatment
procedures:   surgically creating a dam  (pharyngeal flap)  or narrowing
the velopharyngeal port;  constructing a  prosthetic appliance such as a
speech bulb; and, speech therapy provided by the speech-language pathologist.   The decision of which prodecure(s)   is appropriate can be made
only after careful consideration for  the child's health and environmen-
tal/social well being.

## Congenital Malformations

Abnormal resonance due  to defects of the pharyngeal wall  is the result
of congenital malformations;  often  accompanying craniofacial malformations.  Defects occurring after birth are usually the result of tumor or
trauma.

Defects of the tongue also may  be congenital or acquired.  Historically, tongue tie, or ANKYLOGLOSSIA, has been related to possible speech
defects,  and physicians would "clip" the lingual frenulum shortly after
birth.  Today, this procedure is not considered necessary.  In fact, the
possibility of scar tissue formation may pose a greater problem than the
shortened frenulum.   The child does not need to protude the tongue outside the mouth  to produce acceptable speech.   Compensatory oral movements by the speaker can minimize the effects of the defect.   Individuals with aglossia,  loss of tongue,  demonstrate  remarkable ability to
make compensatory strategies to speak intelligibly.

Hypertrophied tonsils may  affect both resonance and  articulation of
children.   The enlargement  of tonsils and adenoidal  tissue may effect
resonance of the oral cavity by changing the shape of the cavity,  i.e.,
narrowing the isthmus of fauces,  and by obstructing the posterior nasal
orifice, resulting in hyponasality.  In addition, the hypertrophied tonsils may cause the child to carry the tongue in a more forward position,
again changing the cavity's shape  and possibly effecting normal articulatory placement of the tongue during speech.

## Dysphagia

DYSPHAGIA  treatment  has increasingly  come  under  the domain  of  the
speech-language pathologist.   Dysphagia refers to disorders of swallowing and can be categorized as:   mechanical dysphasia;  paralytical dysphagia; and pseudobulbar dysphagia.

Mechanical dysphasia involves those conditions, usually the result of
surgery or trauma, that prevents the person from moving food to the back
of the mouth.   Paralysis that affects  the swallowing muscles is due to
lesion or trauma to the cranial nerves or brain stem.  Pseudobulbar dysphagia involves the inability to initiate  the movement of swallowing or
coordinate the muscles properly to swallow.

Management generally involves teaching the patient the isolated steps in swallowing by using stimuli  of various textures,  temperatures,  and tastes.   The patient proceeds from a  reflexive act to volitional swallowing.

## Teeth

The role of teeth in good speech  production has been debated for years. The controversy  stems from a lack  of solid evidence to  substantiate a relationship  between  deviant structures  and articulation  disorders. Some individuals, with what might appear as severe oral structure anomalies, are capable of normal speech.   And,  individuals with no apparent structural defects sometimes have severe articulatory problems.

As a general rule,   it can be assumed that both  children and adults adjust the action of their tongue and  lips to compensate for missing or malaligned teeth.   It has been observed, however, that adults,  such as those with ill-fitting dentures,   may have greater difficulty adjusting to  changes in  the oral  cavity  than children  with dental  anomalies. Young children missing  the upper front incisors are  usually capable of producing acceptable sounds (phonemes).   The role of the speech-language pathologist is to assess  on a case by case basis  the effects of faulty tooth position or dental plate fit.

Tooth malalignment may, for example,  have considerable effect on jaw position, resulting in articulation defects, but may also cause abnormal occlusion.   Occlusal problems will be  discussed in Chapter Five.   Six terms are commonly used to discribe  tooth positions that may create jaw disturbances or sound distortions:

- Axiversion — Improper inclination of the tooth on its long axis.
- Distoversion — Tilting backward or away from midline.
- Infraversion — The failure of the tooth to erupt fully.
- Labioversion — Tilting of the tooth toward the lips.
- Linguoversion — Tilting of the tooth toward the tongue.
- Supraversion — The eruption of a tooth beyond its normal height.

## Glossary

aspiration:     The explosion of air that may accompany stop plosive
     release.

assimilation:     A process of articulation by which individual speech
     sounds become more like those around them.

cognate:     A pair of sounds, identical in place and manner of articula-
     tion, which differ only in presence of absence of voicing.

CPI:     Congenital palatopharyngeal incompetence.

cul-de-sac:     A cavity closed at one end.

diastema:     Abnormally wide spacing between teeth.

dysphagia:     A disorder of swallowing resulting from a lesion of the
     cranial nerves or brain stem.

formant:     A band of resonant energy.

macroglossia:     Abnormally large tongue.

microglossia:     Abnormally small tongue.

open bite:     A clinical condition which results from the lack of normal
     overbite (upper incisors cover the lower incisors).

Passavant's pad:     A ridge projecting from the posterior pharyngeal at
     the level of the horizontal plane of the hard palate, created by
     the hyper contraction of the superior constrictor muscle.

phone:     A particular speech sound.

phoneme:     A group of phones that function in a language to signal a
     difference in meaning.

prosthesis:     An artificial substitute for a missing part.

rhinolalia aperta:     Refers to hyponasality because of the lack of
     patency.

rhinolalia clausa:     Hyponasality or cul-de-sac resonance due to clo-
     sure of the nares.

segment:     A single speech sound, or phone.

torus palatinus:     Benign malformation of medial palatal ridge, which
     appears as a cartilaginous outgrowth.

vocalic:    Refers to a vowel or having vowel-like quality.

# References

Bzock, K.R. (Ed.) (1979).  Communicative disorders related to cleft lip and palate (2nd ed.).  Boston: Little, Brown.

Darley, F. L., Aronson, A. E., & Brown, J. R. (1975).  Motor speech disorders.  Philadelphia: Saunders.

Lass, N. J., McReynolds, L. V., Northern, R. L., & Yoder, D. E.  (1982).  Speech, language, and hearing.  Philadelphia: Saunders.

Mackay, I. (1978).  Introducing practical phonetics.  Boston: Little, Brown.

Mason, R. M. (1973).  Preventing speech disorders following adenoidectomy by preoperative examination.  Clinical Pediatrics, 12, 405-414.

Mason, R.M. and Grandstaff, H. (1970).  Evaluating the velopharyngeal mechanism in hypernasal speakers.  Speech, Language, Hearing Services in the Schools, 4, 26-34.

Zimmerman, J. E., & Oder, L. A. (1981).  Swallowing dysfunction in acutely ill patients.  Physical Therapy, 12, 1755-1763.

# Chapter 5
# Articulation — Skull and Facial Structures

Like mechanisms discussed in Chapter Four, the complex bony network comprising the skull and facial region are important to resonation and articulation. By the action of these structures emotions are expressed, characteristic resonance is imparted to the voice, and precise articulation is possible.

## 5.1 Facial Skeleton

1.  The MANDIBLE (unpaired) forms the lower jaw (Figure 56).

    a.  The corpus, or body, of the mandible is roughly horseshoe shaped.

        i.   This arch is made solid at the ventral midline by the MANDIBULAR SYMPHYSIS.

        ii.  The upper border of the corpus anchors the teeth.

    b.  The RAMI of the mandible extend upward from the posterior parts of the corpus.

        i.    Each is a quadralateral sheet of bone whose superior margin carries two prominent projections.

        ii.   The anterior projection is called the CORANOID process.

        iii.  The posterior projection is the CONDYLOID process.

              1) This process ends in a slight knob called the CAPITULUM.

              2) The capitulum fits into the mandibular fossa of the temporal bone.

2.  The MAXILLA is an irregular bone, forming what is commonly called the upper jaw. It can be divided into five regions (Figure 57)

    a.  The CORPUS is large, quadrangular, and hollow.

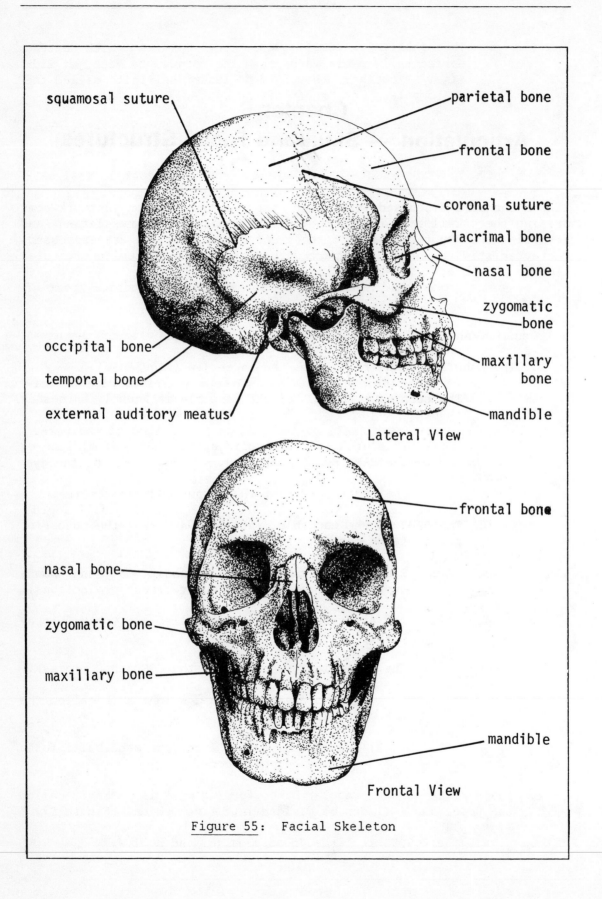

Lateral View

Frontal View

Figure 55:  Facial Skeleton

b.  The PALATINE PROCESS, are bony "plates" which extend horizontally medialward from the corpus to meet at midline. Together they form a functional unit called the "hard palate" or "roof" of the mouth.

c.  The ALVEOLAR PROCESS is a convex arch which extends downward from the corpus into which the teeth are embedded.

d.  The ZYGOMATIC PROCESS extends from the upper lateral margin of the corpus. It joins the zygomatic bone.

e.  The FRONTAL PROCESS ascends to join the frontal bone.

3.  PALATINE bones are irregular "L" shaped bones (Figure 58).

a.  Their horizontal aspects form the most posterior part of the "hard palate".

b.  The vertical extension forms the lateral wall of the nasal cavity.

c.  The superior portion contributes to the floor of the orbital cavity of the eye.

4.  NASAL bones are two small plates forming the bridge of the nose.

5.  LACRIMAL bones form, in part, the medial-anterior wall of the eye orbital cavity.

6.  The VOMER bone is the inferior-posterior part of the nasal septum which divides the nasal cavities.

7.  The INFERIOR NASAL CONCHAE form the inferior part of the lateral nasal walls. They are often described as having a "scroll-like" appearance.

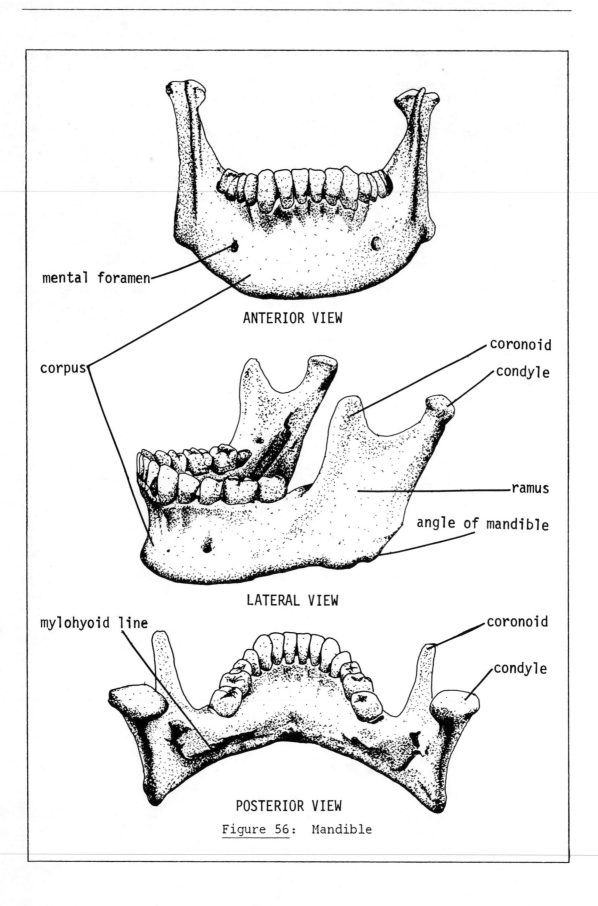

mental foramen

ANTERIOR VIEW

corpus

coronoid

condyle

ramus

angle of mandible

LATERAL VIEW

mylohyoid line

coronoid

condyle

POSTERIOR VIEW

Figure 56: Mandible

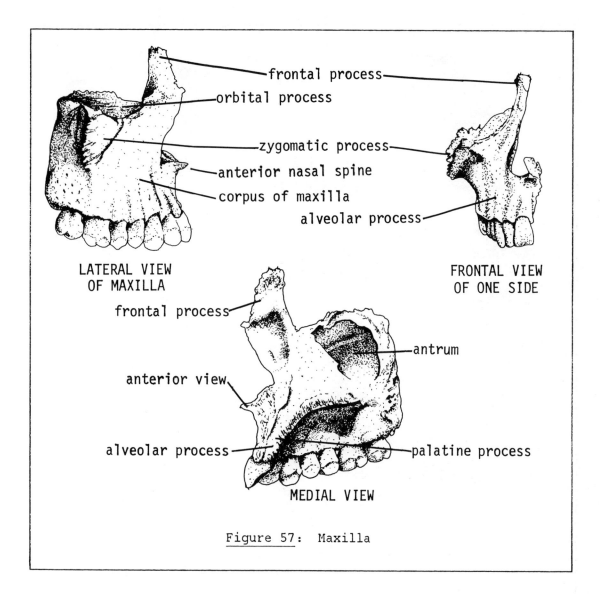

frontal process
orbital process
zygomatic process
anterior nasal spine
corpus of maxilla
alveolar process

LATERAL VIEW
OF MAXILLA

FRONTAL VIEW
OF ONE SIDE

frontal process

antrum

anterior view

alveolar process

palatine process

MEDIAL VIEW

Figure 57:  Maxilla

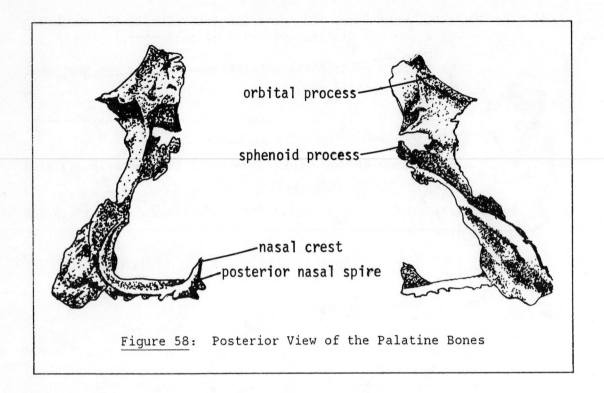

Figure 58:   Posterior View of the Palatine Bones

## 5.2 Cranial Skeleton

The CRANIAL SKELETON is made up of eight bones (Figure 55).

1.   The SPHENOIDAL bone is a "wing" shaped plate which forms part of
     the base of the brain case (Figure 59).

     a.   The lateral and medial pterygoid processes extend downward
          on either side from the GREATER and LESSER WINGS.

     b.   The HAMULAR process is a small projection extending from
          the medial pterygoid plate.

2.   The ETHMOIDAL bone lies deep in the facial skull and helps to
     bound both the nasal cavities and the eye sockets (Figure 60).

     a.   The SUPERIOR and MIDDLE TURBINATE BONES located on the
          lateral nasal wall are parts of the ethmoidal.

     b.   The PERPENDICULAR PLATE of ethmoidal also forms part of
          the nasal septum.

3.   The FRONTAL bone is an unpaired bone forming the "forehead".

4. The TEMPORAL bone forms the anterior-lateral wall of the brain case. There are two distinctive areas of this bone.

    a. The MASTOID process is a thick knob of bone on the lower and outer part of this bone.

    b. The STYLOID is a narrow finger of bone which extends downward and forward.

5. The PARIETAL bones form the greater part of the posterior-lateral and top of the cranial skull.

6. The OCCIPITAL bone is a single large bone forming the posterior aspect of the cranium.

Sinuses

The SINUSES are cavities within the bones of the skull.

1. The FRONTAL sinuses (paired) are located in the frontal bone. They are situated just above the root of the nose.

    a. They are variable in size and divided into separate cavities by a septum, which frequently deviates from the midline.

    b. They open into the nasal cavities below by means of a narrow naso-frontal duct.

2. The MAXILLARY sinuses, or antrum (paired), are the largest of the sinuses and are situated in the maxillary bone. They lie immediately lateral to the nasal cavity.

    a. Their base corresponds to the lateral wall of the nasal cavity.

    b. The sides of the cavities are formed by the orbit and by both the anterior and posterior surfaces of the maxilla.

    c. The one or two openings which lead into the nose are sometimes higher than the sinus floor, causing drainage difficulties and resulting in the feeling of pressure or pain.

3. The ETHMOIDAL sinuses (paired) consist of a series of hollow intercommunicating cells situated between the upper part of the nasal cavity and the orbit of the eye.

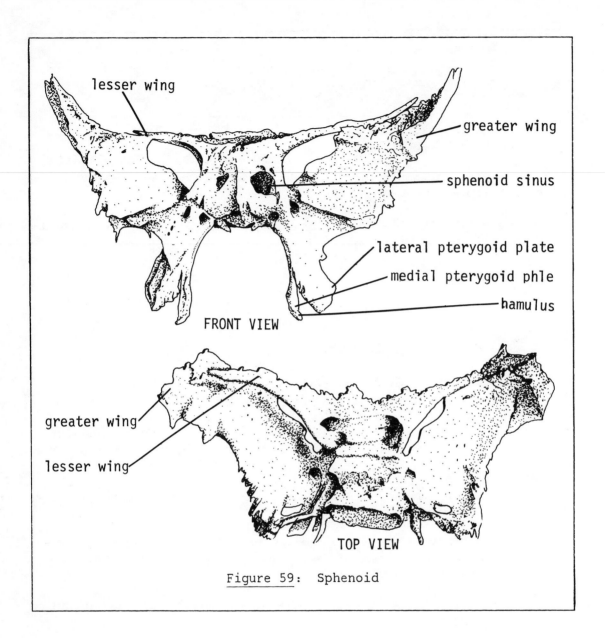

lesser wing

greater wing

sphenoid sinus

lateral pterygoid plate

medial pterygoid phle

hamulus

FRONT VIEW

greater wing

lesser wing

TOP VIEW

Figure 59:  Sphenoid

a.  The cavities are  formed by both the walls  of the ethmoid
and by surrounding bone structures.

b.  Each cavity communicates with the corresponding nasal cavity by means of three or more openings.

4.  The SPHENOIDAL SINUS (unpaired) lies within the body of the sphenoidal bone,  being situated  immediately behind  and above  the
nasal cavities.

a.  It is above and a little anterior to the naso-pharynx.

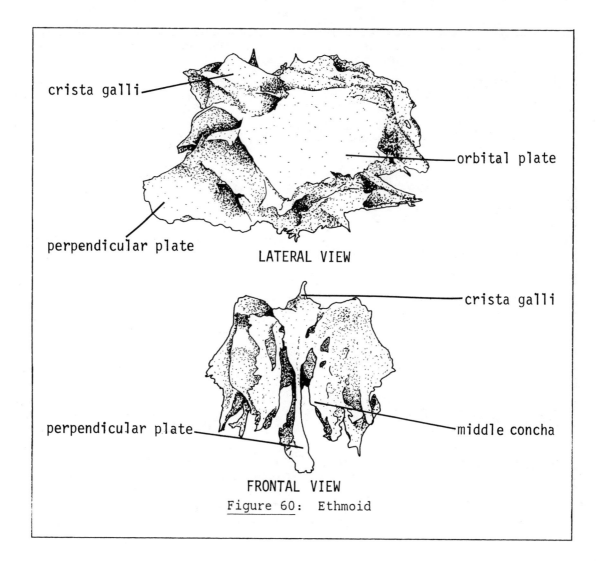

crista galli

orbital plate

perpendicular plate

LATERAL VIEW

crista galli

perpendicular plate

middle concha

FRONTAL VIEW
Figure 60:  Ethmoid

b.  On each  side a  duct connects  it with  the corresponding
nasal cavity.

Nose

The nose is made up of two  cavities separated by bones and cartilage
tissue.

1.  The NASAL SEPTUM (unpaired)  is  a medially-placed vertical sheet
of  bone and  cartilage which  separates the  two nasal  cavities
(Figure 61).

a.  Its anterior portion is cartilaginous.  The posterior part is formed by the vomer bone and the perpendicular plate of the ethmoidal bone.

b.  The septum often deviates anteriorly to the right side.

c.  On the lateral wall of each cavity are found orifices communicating with the frontal,  maxillary, ethmoidal,  and sphenoidal sinuses.

d.  The lateral  walls of the  nasal cavities are  complex and irregular, being formed by parts of various skull bones.

2.  The TURBINATE bones, or CONCHAE (paired) are thin,  curled ledges projecting into  the nasal cavity  from the lateral  wall (Figure 62).

a.  The SUPERIOR  TURBINATE,  the smallest of  the turbinates, lies on the superior posterior part of the lateral wall.

b.  The  MIDDLE TURBINATE,  nearly twice  the  length of  the superior, is situated below the latter and extends farther forward.

c.  The INFERIOR TURBINATE is the  inferior and largest of the turbinates.

d.  The upper two  pairs of turbinates are formed  by the ethmoidal bone,  while the inferior turbinates  are separate bones.

e.  The turbinates are covered by mucous membrane, that serves to filter and condition the air carried into the lungs.

3.  Because the nasal cavities are irregularly shaped,  the nose acts as a multiple resonator.


Facial Expression

Muscles of  facial expression act upon  the mouth slit.   These muscles originate either from bone or superficial  fascia and insert into mucosa of the skin or interdigitate with other facial muscles (Figure 63).

1.  The lips border the  mouth slit and have a red  area known as the VERMILION ZONE.

a.  The lips extend beyond the vermilion zone.

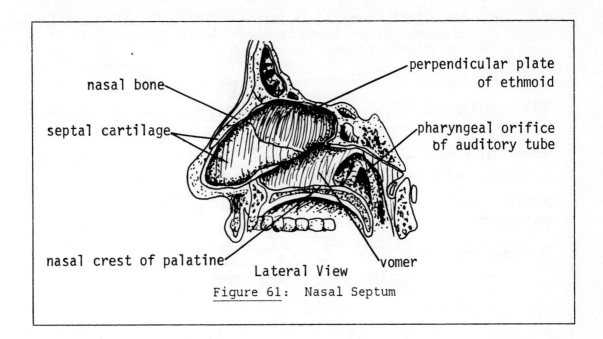

Lateral View

Figure 61:  Nasal Septum

   b.  The lips are  composed of four layers  known as integument
       (external skin), muscle, glands, and internal mucosa.

2.  A principal muscle of lip movement is the ORBICULARIS ORIS.

   a.  This singular  complex muscle  is a  circle of  concentric
       fibers surrounding the lips.

   b.  Numerous facial  muscles insert  into the  border of  this
       muscle.

   c.  The action of the orbicularis oris is to close lips.

3.  The primary  elevators of  the upper  lip are  the LEVATOR  LABII
    SUPERIORIS (paired)  muscles.   Each muscle  pair has three heads
    that originate from  the maxillae and zygomatic  bones and insert
    into the orbicularis oris.

   a.  The smallest  of the heads  is the ZYGOMATICUS  MINOR that
       arises from the zygomatic bone.

   b.  The middle INFRAORBITAL HEAD orginates  under the orbit of
       the eye.

   c.  The ALA NASI (angular)  HEAD orginates on the frontal pro-
       cess of the maxilla.   In addition to aiding in the eleva-
       tion of the lip, this muscle serves to flare the nostril.

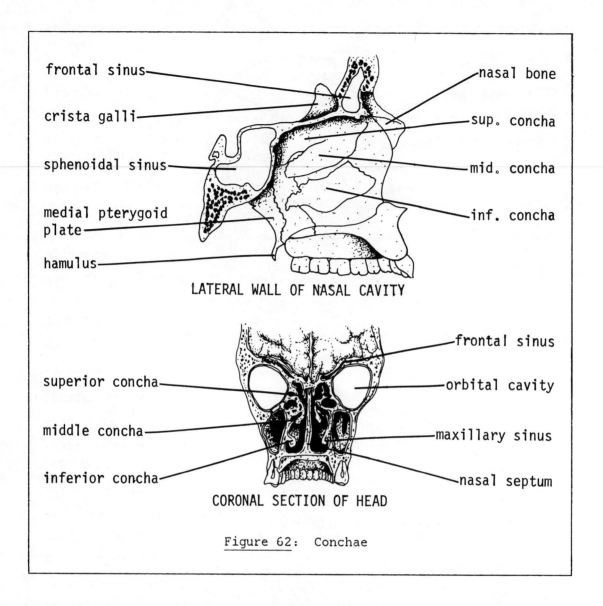

LATERAL WALL OF NASAL CAVITY

CORONAL SECTION OF HEAD

Figure 62:  Conchae

4.  The ZYGOMATICUS MAJOR (paired)  are long slender muscles that lie at an angle to the side of the face.

    a.  These muscles originate on the zygomatic process and insert into the orbicularis oris at the corner of the mouth.

    b.  The function of these muscles is to pull the corner of the mouth to the side and upward (smile).

5.  RISORIUS (paired) muscles are variable in humans and, therefore, may or may not be developed.

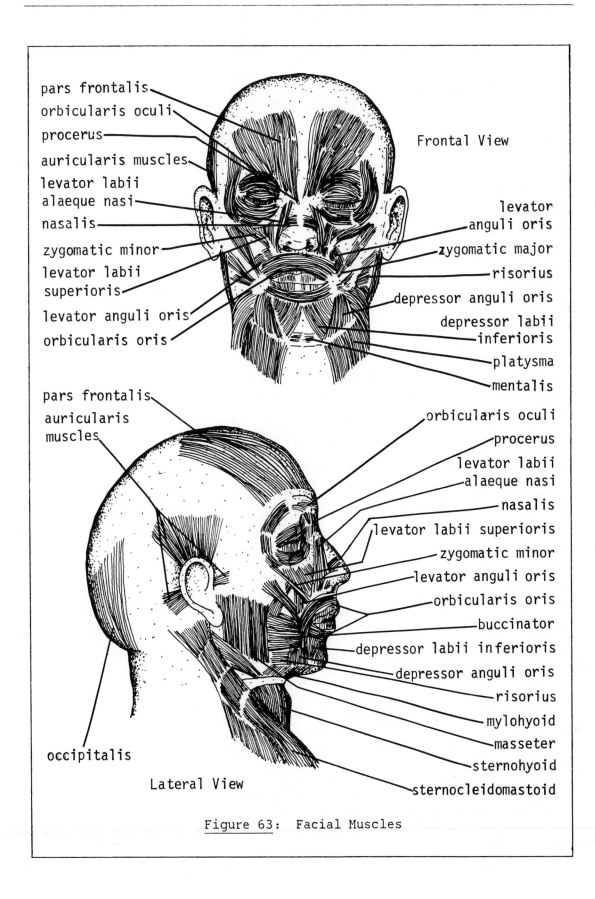

pars frontalis
orbicularis oculi
procerus
auricularis muscles
levator labii
alaeque nasi
nasalis
zygomatic minor
levator labii
superioris
levator anguli oris
orbicularis oris

Frontal View

levator
anguli oris
zygomatic major
risorius
depressor anguli oris
depressor labii
inferioris
platysma
mentalis

pars frontalis
auricularis
muscles

orbicularis oculi
procerus
levator labii
alaeque nasi
nasalis
levator labii superioris
zygomatic minor
levator anguli oris
orbicularis oris
buccinator
depressor labii inferioris
depressor anguli oris
risorius
mylohyoid
masseter
sternohyoid
sternocleidomastoid

occipitalis

Lateral View

Figure 63:  Facial Muscles

a.  The origin is the fascia covering the masseter muscles
    that inserts into the angle of the mouth.

b.  These muscles aid in drawing the corner of the mouth back
    as in smiling.

6.  The LEVATOR ANGULI ORIS (paired) are small muscles that are also
    known as the CANINE muscles located above the canine teeth.

    a.  These muscles originate from the canine fossa of the max-
        illa and insert into the corner of the mouth.

    b.  Their function is to elevate the corners of the mouth.

7.  The DEPRESSOR LABII INFERIORIS muscles (paired), located beneath
    the lip, are small muscles sometimes known as the QUADRATUS LABII
    INFERIOR.

    a.  These muscles originate on the mandible either side of
        midline and insert along the midline of the lip.

    b.  The muscles pull the lip down and away from the alveolar
        ridge.

    c.  The DEPRESSOR ANGULI ORIS (triangularis) muscles (paired)
        are located lateral to the depressor labii inferioris.

        i.   They originate on the mandible.

        ii.  Most of the fibers of these muscles insert at the
             lower angle of the mouth; however, some fibers con-
             tinue around to insert in the upper corner of the
             mouth.

        iii. These muscles draw the angle of the mouth downward.

8.  Also located on the mandible are the MENTALIS muscles (paired).

    a.  These small groups of muscle fibers originate on the man-
        dible and insert into the superficial mucosa covering the
        chin.

    b.  The action of the muscles is to protrude the lower lip and
        "dimple" the chin.

9.  There are two pairs of INCISIVIS muscles; the superior and
    inferior.

    a.  The SUPERIOR MUSCLES originate at the canine eminence of
        the maxilla and insert into the orbicularis oris at the
        upper corner of the mouth.

b.  The SUPERIOR INCISIVIS MUSCLES draw  the upper lip upward
and medially.

c.  The INFERIOR INCISIVIS  MUSCLES draw the lower  lip downward and medially.

10.  The PLATYSMA (unpaired)  is a  thin superficial sheet  of muscle
that primarily covers the anterior-lateral neck region.

a.  It orginates from the superficial mucosa of the clavicular
area and  inserts on  the mandible from  the angle  of the
ramus on one side to the other.

b.  In speech this muscle probably serves to pull the mandible
downward and  the corner of  the mouth angle  downward and
lateralward.

## Lateral Cheek Wall

The muscles that  form the lateral cheek wall are  called the BUCCINATOR
(paired).    They can  be  regarded as  the  forward extensions of  the
superior pharyngeal constrictor muscle of the pharynx.

1.  These muscles originate from three  areas:   the alveolar process
of the maxilla, the mandible, and the pterygomandibular raphe.

a.  The  PTERYGOMANDIBULAR LIGAMENT  runs on  a vertical  plan
from the hamulus process of  the medial pterygoid plate to
the mylohyoid line of the mandible.

b.  The structure of attachment  separates the buccinator from
the superior pharyngeal constrictor muscle.

2.  The insertion of  the buccinators is the orbicularis  oris at the
upper and lower corners of the mouth.

3.  The buccinator muscles compress the "cheeks" serving to hold food
between the teeth and to pull the corners of the mouth laterally.

## Nose Structure

The bones  and cartilage that  make up the  scaffolding of the  nose are
covered by three paired muscles and a single muscle.

1.  The PROCERUS (unpaired) muscle covers the ridge of the nose.

      a.   The muscle originates along the  lower margin of the nasal bones.

      b.   The fibers course upward to insert  into the mucosa of the skin between the eyebrows.

      c.   The procerus draws the angle of  the eyebrow down and creates horizontal wrinkles above the bridge of the nose giving a "quizzical" appearance.

2.   The ANTERIOR and POSTERIOR DILATOR NARES (paired)  flare the ala (wing) of the nose, enlarging the nostril.

      a.   Each anterior dilator  originates on the edge  of the lateral cartilage and inserts into the mucosa of the skin.

      b.   Each posterior  dilator arises  from the  maxilla and  the sesamoid cartilage of  the nose and inserts  into the skin covering the alar cartilages.

      c.   By enlarging the  nostril these muscles may  allow greater air intake.  For  facial expression they contribute  to a look of anger.

3.   The DEPRESSOR  SEPTI (paired),  also called  the DEPRESSOR  ALAE NASI,  serve to constrict the nares,   decreasing the size of the nostril.

      a.   These muscles  originate from  the incisive  fossa of  the maxilla.

      b.   They insert into the lower margin of the alae of the nose.

4.   The NASALIS (paired) muscles  also arise from  the area  of the incisive fossa of  the maxilla and course upward  and medially to the upper margin (ridge) of the nasal cartilage.

      a.   At the  median ridge  of the  nasal cartilage  the nasalis muscles from  one side  interdigitate with  their opposite muscles on the other side.

      b.   These muscles  serve to  depress the  nasal cartilage  and compress (narrow) the alae.

## Eye and Scalp

Facial expression is also controlled by  muscles around the eye and muscles of the scalp.

1. The ORBICULARIS OCULI (paired) are sphincteric muscles that surround the eye socket in concentric rings.  Each of these muscles has two parts.

    a.  The ORBITAL part orginates at the  medial angle of the eye by the palpebral ligament.

        i.  The  fibers go  around the  lid  forming the  outer rings of the orbicularis oculi.

        ii.  The orbital fibers draw the eyebrows down.

    b.  The PALPEBRAL part  originates from the same  point as the orbital to form the inside ring of fibers.

        i.  These  fibers insert  into the  corner  of the  eye socket.

        ii.  Their position  serves to form  the fascia  for the lacrimal sac and functions to compress the sac.

        iii.  It also acts to close the eyelid.

2. Superficial muscles  of the eye  that draw the  eyebrows downward and  medially,  as  when  frowning,  are called  the CORRUGATOR SUPERCILII (paired).

    a.  The muscles arise from the  superciliary arch on the frontal bone  and insert into the  skin of the  medial eyebrow region.

    b.  When these muscles contract, vertical wrinkles are created between the eyebrows.

3. The LEVATOR PALPEBRAE SUPERIORIS (paired)  are muscles that raise the eyelid.

    a.  These muscles originate at the superior margin of the back of the eye socket.

    b.  The fibers run downward to insert  into the medial edge of the upper lid called the TARSAL PLATE.

4. The SCALP  MUSCLES move the scalp  back and forth  by alternating contractions.

    a.  The OCCIPITALIS (paired) originates on  the back  of the skull and inserts into the deepest layer of the scalp, the EPICRANIUS (aponeurotic tissue).

b. The occipitalis joins the FRONTALIS (paired) at the epi-
   cranius. From this point the frontalis courses forward to
   insert into the skin of the forehead.

c. The frontalis raises the eyebrows and creates horizontal
   forehead wrinkles.

## Mastication

The muscles of MASTICATION are facial muscles that have a specialized
function. These muscles insert on the mandible, and are concerned with
chewing and biting.

1. The MASSETER (paired) muscles arise from two areas (Figure 64).

   a. Superficially these muscles arise from the lower border of
      the zygomatic arch.

   b. Fibers also originate on the posterior-medial surface of
      the zygomatic arch.

   c. From these points of origin the muscles run downward to
      insert along the ramus of the mandible from the condyloid
      region to the angle.

   d. Upon contraction these muscles close the jaw by elevating
      and drawing the mandible back.

   e. Tension in these muscles can be felt by clenching the
      teeth.

2. Closely associated with the masseter are the MEDIAL PTERYGOID
   (internal pterygoid muscles) that are located deep to the ramus
   of the mandible (Figure 65).

   a. These muscles originate from the lateral pterygoid plate
      of the sphenoid, pyramidal process of the palatine bone
      and tuberosity of the maxilla.

   b. Coursing downward, laterally and posteriorly, the fibers
      insert into the lower margin of the medial surface of the
      mandible, near the insertion of the masseter.

   c. Collectively, the medial pterygoid and masseter form a
      sling that holds the mandible -- the MANDIBULAR SLING.

   d. The action of the medial pterygoid is both to raise the
      mandible and to protrude it.

3. The (paired)  LATERAL PTERYGOID (external pterygoid),  together with the  digastric and mylohyoid  muscles (discussed  in Chapter Three) serve to depress the mandible.

    a. The origin of the lateral pterygoid muscles is the lateral pterygoid plate and greater wing of the sphenoid.

    b. From these two points,  the  fibers run backward to insert into the neck of the mandibular condyle and articular disc at the temporal-mandibular joint.

    c. Together these  muscles protrude  the mandible  and consequently aid in depressing and/or opening the jaw.  By acting in an alternating fashion  they move the mandible from side to side (chewing).

4. The TEMPORALIS  (paired) muscles are  shaped like a  fan (Figure 66).

    a. The broad extension of fibers  originate from the temporal fossa on the skull.

    b. The fibers converge  to insert on the  coronoid process of the mandible.

    c. They serve  to close the  jaw by retracting  and elevating the mandible.

    d. The temporalis muscles can be felt by clenching the jaw.

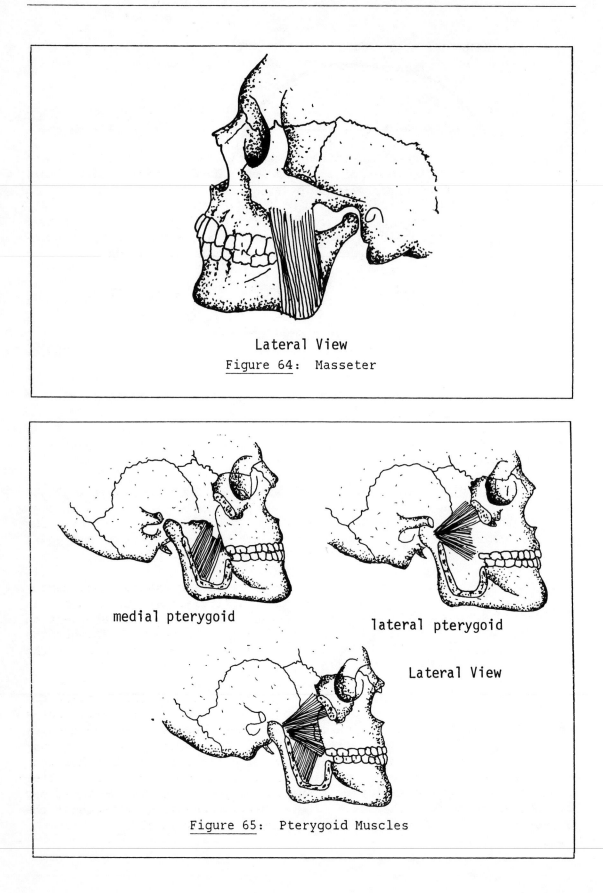

Lateral View
Figure 64:  Masseter

medial pterygoid

lateral pterygoid

Lateral View

Figure 65:  Pterygoid Muscles

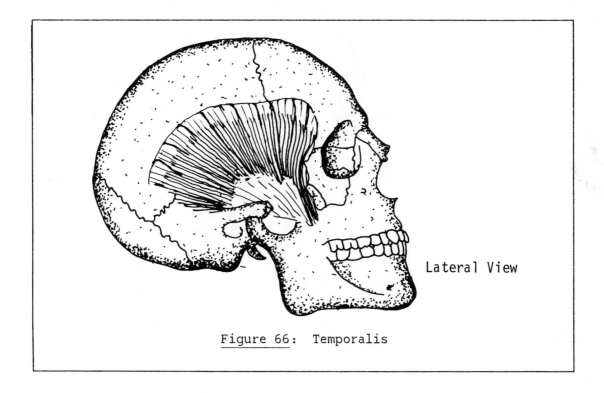

Lateral View

Figure 66:  Temporalis

## 5.3 Physiological Implications -- Jaw and Lips

Since the 1970's extensive research has been done investigating the relationship of mandibular movement and connected speech.    Until that time the jaw was, at best, considered a secondary articulator.    The early phonetic theories were concerned with tongue position and vowel production, with little, if any, consideration of jaw position.

Today speech physiology studies have provided information that demonstrates that jaw movement influences other articulators, but, also, is influenced by those articulators.   Movement of the lips is dependent on jaw position; so too, is the tongue affected by the jaw.   The higher the tongue tip positon required to produce a phoneme, the more closed is the jaw.   The jaw never closes completely during connected speech.

Studies have been conducted to determine which muscles function for jaw closure during speech, and to what extent each muscle participates in this maneuver.   Based primarily on studies that examined the muscles of mastication those muscles responsible for jaw closure are the masseter, temporalis, and medial pterygoid.   The lateral pterygoid has traditionally been viewed as a muscle used to open the jaw.   This latter assumption has been questioned.   Anatomically the lateral pterygoid may better serve to close the jaw.   There is evidence, also, to suggest the extent of its activity may be variable between individuals.

The medial pterygoid seems to be the most active muscle during speech. Again, however, there is considerable variance between speakers, suggesting that for different individuals, different combinations of muscle function are appropriate for normal speech production. The dynamic relationship between the jaw muscles for speech is not fully understood. The effect each muscle has on the action of the other muscle(s), including mechanical factors and neurological interrelationships, needs to be studied further.

Lip movements have typically been associated with the degree of lip rounding for the production of vowels. As a general rule, as the dorsum of the tongue moves back and upward to produce a vowel, a greater degree of lip rounding is evident (contrasting the degree of lip rounding and tongue position during the production of the vowels /i/ and /u/).

Lip rounding has been used as a marker in studies of COARTICULATION. Coarticulation is the simultaneous "overlap" of two or more speech sounds. During speech several phonemes are produced in the same or similar articulatory gestures. For the isolated production of /t/, /r/, /u/, lip rounding does not occur until the production of /u/. When the phones are combined to form /tru/, lip rounding occurs at the beginning of the /t/ phoneme. This type of lip organization lends support to the notion that spoken words are divided neurologically rather than simply divided into discrete acoustic segments.

Neuromuscular events involved in coarticulation, as measured by lip rounding, are not bound by a specific phonatory event. A popular model that has been used to explain the anticipatory nature of coarticulation is the LOOK-AHEAD (scanning) MODEL. This model explains the anticipatory articulation gesture (e.g. lip rounding occurring at the beginning of the /t/ in the work /tru/) by suggesting that a specific phonemic feature is initiated when a scanning device determines that the movement is possible. When gestures occur that are contradictory to the target feature, the motor system command will not occur until the antagonistic gesture has been articulated.

There has been research that suggests that the look-ahead model may not present a complete explanation of coarticulation. Biomechanical conditions exist that influence the scanning device's "decision-making". When the first vowel is biomechanically antagonistic to rounding (e.g. /i/), and the target feature is /u/, then lip activity will begin and end with greater force than if the initial syllable was in a neutral position for /a/. Therefore, for the lips which are unique articulators in that they involve both agonistic and antagonistic action, biomechanical conditions control the anticipatory gesture toward the phoneme target even though it is antagonistic to the feature being sought by the scanner.

For other articulators, such as the velum, whose action is not in conflict with itself, the look-ahead model may still be the best explanation of coarticulation gestures. The jaw, tongue, and velum anticipatory action  for vowels may  be confined to  vowel-consonant-vowel (VCV) utterances rather than the more complex units of VCCCV.

Usually the upper  lip and lower lip move in  unison.  However,  the extent of movement varies.  If there is increased movement in one, there is a decrease in  the other.  The lower lip is  greatly affected by jaw movement and takes a greater role in sound production (e.g.  labiodental sounds).

## 5.4 Clinical Applications

To appreciate clinical conditions that affect the facial skeleton, it is helpful to understand the growth patterns of the face and skull.  Growth of the facial  bones is in a  forward and downward direction  that moves away from the cranial base.  This "direction" of growth is due to actual growth  of bone  on the  posterior and  superior aspects  of the  facial bones.   The growth of the skeletal structures is not the result of bone growing proportionally  in all  directions.   That is,  the  difference between the mandible of an adult and a  child is not merely one of over-all enlargement (Figure 67).

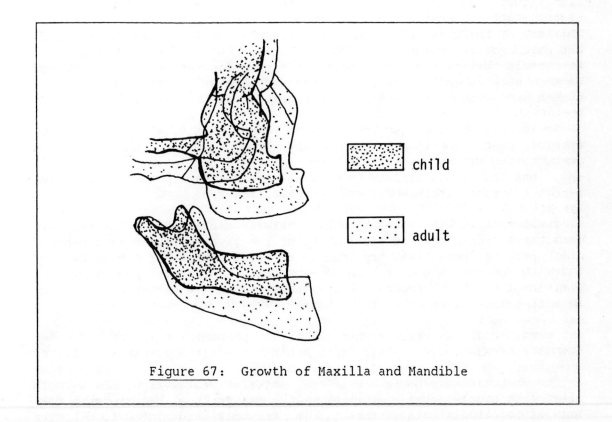

Figure 67:  Growth of Maxilla and Mandible

Rather, growth and "remodeling" of a structure takes place by a process of DEPOSITION and RESORPTION. Deposition is the term used to describe new deposits of bone tissue on skeletal structures. Resorption is the process of "sloughing" bony tissue. Actual mandibular growth and shaping is a result of this dynamic adding and subtracting process. The maxilla follows a similar pattern as the mandible: superior and posterior growth results in an anterior and inferior direction of growth. The facial skeleton is also dependent upon the influences of the muscles of the face, tongue, and teeth.

To help understand the direction of facial growth, consider the head of the infant as an egg positioned so that its oblong appearance is on the horizontal axis. Comparatively, the head of the adult can be likened to an egg in an upright position supported on its narrowest end.

The skull follows a different development sequence. During the first two years of life the cranium triples in volume and by age ten an individual's cranium will be approximately 90 per cent of its adult size. After the first year the facial region grows faster than the skull.

There are numerous anomalies affecting craniofacial structures. A discussion of specific syndromes is beyond the scope of this text but, what is important to understand is the effect such structural deviations may have on speech. It is tempting to state that the gross malocclusion, tooth malalignments, missing teeth, absence of structures or organs, and tissue deviations would have a direct effect on speech. This is not the case. Disorders of articulation, resonance, hearing, and psychosocial problems do occur, but not with any direct correlation. A specific defect may not result in a specific articulation problem. Factors such as emotion or faulty learning play an important role in the speech and language of persons with craniofacial anomalies.

It is the job of the speech language pathologist to assess the influence of speech function to the deviant structure. The therapist, in consultation with professionals from medicine, dentistry, and psychology, has the responsibility to evaluate this speech pattern and recommend appropriate therapeutic speech rehabilitation.

There is a necessary relationship between dentition and the mandible to achieve proper closure (occlusion) of the jaws. Proper alignment of the upper and lower teeth provides an efficient surface for mastication, allowing for normal dental arch development, and correct positioning of individual teeth. Abnormal occlusion may be due to either abnormal jaw development or abnormal tooth position.

Normal occlusion results when the first permanent molar on the upper jaw is approximately one-half tooth behind the first permanent molar of the lower jaw. It is possible for an individual to have normal molar occlusion but have a deviation in the anterior dental arch, as seen in some cleft palate cases. Further, a normal occlusal relationship does not insure normal tooth alignment. A commonly used system to describe occlusal relationship is ANGLE'S classification (Figure 68).

1.  Class I:    Normal molar relationship  but having  abnormal tooth alignment (neutrocclusion).

2.  Class II:    The mandibular molar  is posterior to normal position (distocclusion).

3.  Class III:    The mandibular molar  is anterior to normal position (mesioccluson).

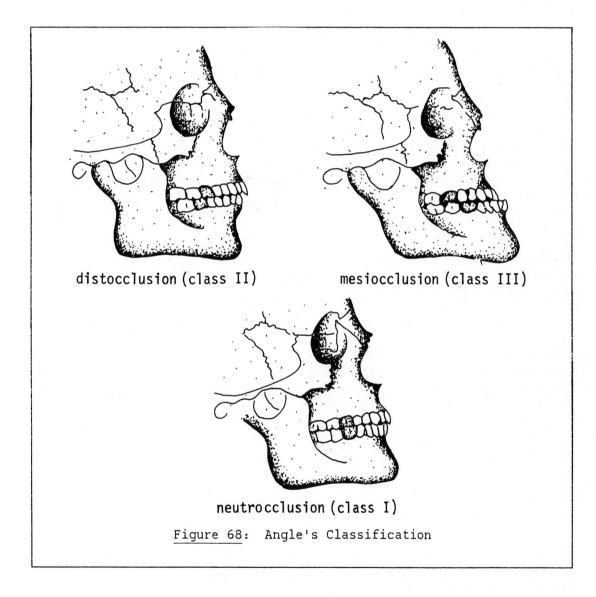

distocclusion (class II)          mesiocclusion (class III)

neutrocclusion (class I)

Figure 68:  Angle's Classification

A clinical condition that has a profound effect on some individuals, and also demonstrates the dynamic relationship between muscles of mastication and the structures of dentition, is TEMPOROMANDIBULAR JOINT syndrome. This condition, seen more in females than males, results in pain or tenderness or decreased joint mobility. The causes of this problem are not clear; hypotheses have included anxiety, dental maloccluson, metabolic and nutritional imbalance. Whatever the cause -- organic or functional -- the effect of one group of muscles and structures may have a profound effect on the others. In many cases x-ray examination of the joint shows no gross abnormality. Diagnosis of this syndrome may be done through evaluation of dental occlusion and by electromyography (EMG) of the muscles of mastication.

The use of x-rays has played an important role in medical and dental science in the diagnosis and treatment of diseases and anomalies; providing records of growth of the bony and soft tissues of the skull and faces; and assessing the functioning of the speech mechanisms.

Two basic radiographic techniques are used to evaluate the structures of the head: fixed lateral x-rays, and motion picture film. The latter process, commonly called cinefluorography, has been used extensively to determine the adequacy of the velopharyngeal mechanism in hypernasal speakers. The cinefluorographic method is usually employed when a study of continuous speech is made and the procedure is accompanied by a sound track recording that can be played back simultaneously with the moton picture.

In recent years fiberoptics and ultrasound have been used as alternatives to x-ray examination. Both procedures can be used to obtain permanent motion picture recording.

Computerization of cephalometric x-rays has added greatly to the accuracy in assessing facial growth. By such techniques, both bone and soft tissue can be analyzed. Accurate evaluative advances have helped to dispel some clinical impressions describing a client as having low set ears, high palatal arch, or wide spread eyes, when, in fact, there has been no documentation for these observations.

## Glossary

ankylosis:    Immobility of a joint.

anomalad:    A malformation together with its subsequently derived structural changes.

biostereometrics:    Contour mapping of various forms.

buccal:    The cheek.

cheilosis:    Fissuring and dry scaling of the vermilion surface of the lips and angles of the mouth.

cinefluorography:    An extension of basic radiological procedures, but the conventional still x-ray is replaced by a motion picture camera.

columella:    The lower margin of the nasal septum.

craniostenosis:    Deformity of the skull due to premature closure of the cranial sutures.  The cranium will grow in the direction of the prematurely closed suture.

hypertelorism:    Abnormally wide spacing between eyes.

malformation:    A primary structural defect that results from localized error or morphogenesis.

micrognathia:    Small (hypoplastic) mandible.

osteology:    The study of bones.

philtrum:    A vertical medline depression extending from the vermilion to the base of the columella of the nose.

ptosis:    Drooping of the upper eyelid.

radiology:    A branch of medical science that deals with the use of radioactive substances and x-rays in the diagnosis and treatment of disease.

roentgen:    A standard international unit of (X-ray) radiation.

# References

Basmajian, J. V. (1977).  Surface anatomy: An instruction manual.
     Baltimore:  Williams & Wilkins.

Clifford, E. (1972).  Psychological aspects of orofacial anomalies:
     Speculation in search of data.  Orofacial Anomalies:  Clinical and
     Research Implications, Proceedings of the Conference.  ASHA
     Reports, 6, 2-29.

Folkins, J. W. (1981).  Muscle activity for jaw closing during speech.
     Journal of Speech Hearing Research, 24, 601-615.

Gorlin, R. J., Pindborg, J. J., & Cohen, M. M. (1976).  Syndromes of the
     head and neck (2nd ed.).  San Francisco: McGraw-Hill.

Moyers, R. E. (1971).  Postnatal development of the orofacial
     musculature.  Patterns of Orofacial Growth and Development,
     Proceedings of the Conference.  ASHA Reports, 6, 38-47.

Peterson-Falzone, S. (1982).  Articulation disorders in orofacial
     anomalies.  In N. J. Lass, V. McReyholds, J. L. Northern, & D. E.
     Yoder (Eds.), Speech, Language, and Hearing:  Vol. II.
     Philadelphia: Saunders.

Zemlin, W. R. (1981).  Speech and hearing science (2nd ed.).  Englewood
     Cliffs, NJ: Prentice Hall.

# Chapter 6
# The Ear and Hearing

The ear is an organ of hearing, presenting a mechanism through which sound waves are conducted and converted into electrical signals. These signals are conveyed to the brain where they are interpreted into meaningful units. Audition is the primary avenue by which language is learned. A distruption in the hearing mechanism may interfere with the normal acquisition of language, and consequently, may result in abnormal oral language expression.

## 6.1 External Ear

The EXTERNAL EAR consists of the auricle (pinna) and the external auditory meatus (canal) (Figure 69).

1. The AURICLE projects from the side of the head.

    a. It is composed of elastic cartilage and fibrous tissue and is divided into seven landmarks that are represented in Figure 69.

    b. The auricle's function is to aid sound localization.

    c. Unlike other animals, humans lack the ability to move the auricle in the attempt to localize sound precisely.

2. The EXTERNAL AUDITORY MEATUS extends from the CONCHA to the TYMPANIC membrane (eardrum), about 2.5 cm in length in the adult male.

    a. It is lined with skin, the outer one-third of which is called the CERUMEN TUBERCLE. This area of the canal contains hair follicles and mucous glands which secrete wax (cerumen).

    b. The medial two-thirds of the canal skin lie immediately over bone and are referred to as the OSSEOUS region.

    c. The auditory meatus is irregular in its path from the concha to the tympanic membrane with the largest diameter near the outside, and the smallest near the tympanic membrane.

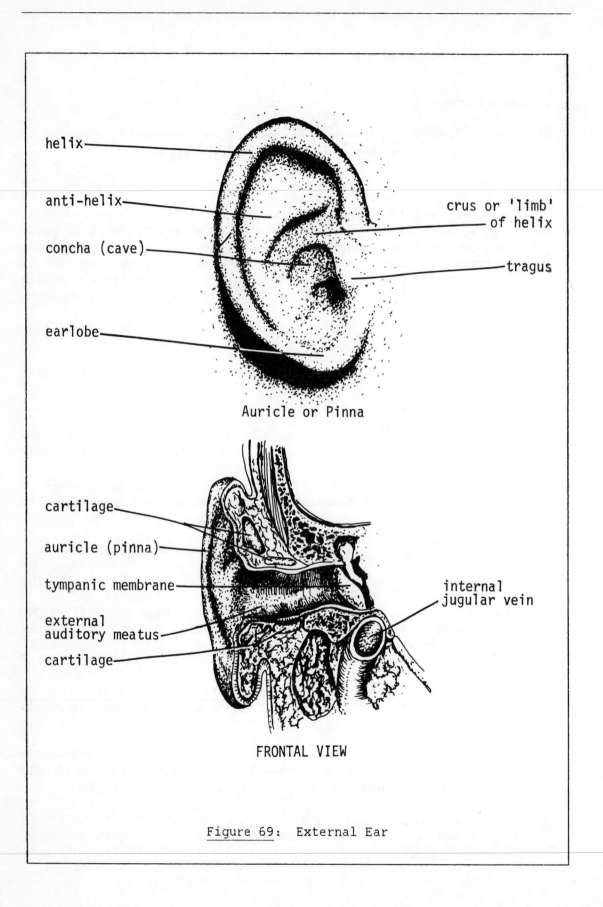

Auricle or Pinna

FRONTAL VIEW

Figure 69:  External Ear

## 6.2 Middle Ear

1. The TYMPANIC membrane slopes forward and inward at about a 55 degree angle in the adult (Figure 70).

    a. A bone of the middle ear (malleus) is attached to the membrane at a point called the UMBO.

    b. The circular membrane is set in a groove and moves with changes in air pressure (sound).

2. The tympanic cavity forms an area that houses the ossicular chain.

    a. Through the floor in this cavity opens the eustachian tube.

    b. Through the eustachian tube the middle ear communicates with the nasopharynx that allows for equalization of air pressure within the middle ear.

3. The OSSICULAR CHAIN transmits vibration of sound from the tympanic membrane to the inner ear. The three bones of the chain are the smallest in the human body (Figure 70).

    a. The MALLEUS joins the tympanic membrane and the incus.

    b. The INCUS joins the malleus and the stapes

    c. The STAPES attaches to the oval window that marks the medial boundary of the middle ear.

4. The medial wall of the middle ear cavity contains the oval window and round window.

    a. The OVAL WINDOW is set in motion by the direct action of the foot-plate of the stapes.

    b. This motion then transfers to fluid in the cochlea of the inner ear.

    c. The ROUND WINDOW acts as a shock absorber to absorb the pressure that moves through the cochlea from the oval window.

5.  Muscles of the Middle Ear

    a.  The TENSOR TYMPANI arises from cartilaginous part of audi-
        tory tube and greater wing of sphenoid bone and inserts on
        malleus.   Action of this muscle  is to tense the tympanic
        membrane by drawing the malleus medially and anteriorly.

    b.  The STAPEDIUS originates on the posterior wall of the cav-
        ity and via a tendon attaches  to the stapes.   The action
        is to pull the stapes posteriorly.

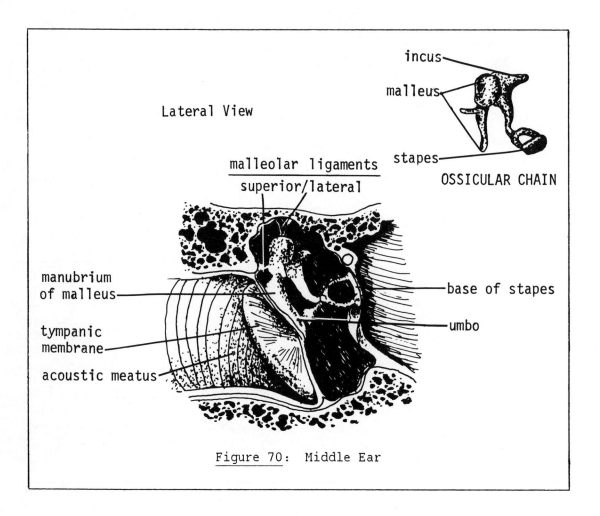

Figure 70:  Middle Ear

## 6.3 Inner Ear

Structure of the Inner Ear

The inner ear is divided into structures for hearing and for equilibrium. Both functions are structurally interconnected by a bony covering (laryrinth), membranous sacs, and tubes.

1. The BONY LABYRINTH has three parts (Figure 71).

    a. The VESTIBULE, which houses the oval window, provides an area for nerves and ducts, an opening for the semicircular canals, and an opening for the cochlea.

    b. The SEMICIRCULAR CANAL is composed of three parts: superior, posterior, and lateral canals.

        i. The superior and posterior canals have a common trunk called the COMMON CRUS.

        ii. Each canal has an enlargement called an AMPULA.

        iii. These lead into the vestibule.

    c. The COCHLEA spirals like a snail's shell, having a base and apex.

        i. This bony canal spirals about 2 1/2 times.

        ii. The cochlea is divided into a SCALA VESTIBULI and a SCALA TYMPANI. The two tracts communicate at the apex via the HELICOTREMA.

        iii. The SCALA VESTIBULI begins at the oval window and the SCALA TYMPANI terminates with the round window.

2. MEMBRANOUS LABYRINTH is connective tissue, filled with endolymph fluid that forms, within the bony labyrinth, four areas (Figure 72).

    a. Within the vestibuli are formed the UTRICLE and SACCULI. The utricle and sacculi contain sensory endings for equilibrium.

        i. The utricle has five openings for the semicircular canal ducts.

        ii. The sacculi connects into the cochlear duct.

    b. The SEMICIRCULAR CANALS conform to the contours of the bony labyrinth.

c. The COCHLEAR DUCT runs the length of the cochlear canal to the apex and is sandwiched between scala vestibuli and scala tympani.

   i. The duct is separated from the scala vestibuli by the VESTIBULAR MEMBRANE.

   ii. The scala tympani is separated from the duct by BASILAR MEMBRANE.

   iii. The duct is the origin of the cochlear nerve.

   iv. The cochlear duct is widened and less stiff as it approaches the apex.

   v. The basilar membrane side of the duct gives rise to the Organ of Corti.

      1) The Organ of Corti includes: three to four rows or outer hair cells and one row of inner hair cells; cells of Ceiter, Claudius and Hansen; the tunnel or corti; and the tectorial membrane.

      2) There approximately 13,500 outer hair cells and 3,500 inner hair cells.

## Fluids of the Inner Ear

The inner ear is filled with two, possibly three, fluids, each of different composition.

1. The bony labyrinth is filled with PERILYMPH which surrounds the membranous labyrinth.

2. The membranous labyrinth contains ENDOLYMPH.

3. Cortilymph is hypothesized to exist in the Organ of Corti.

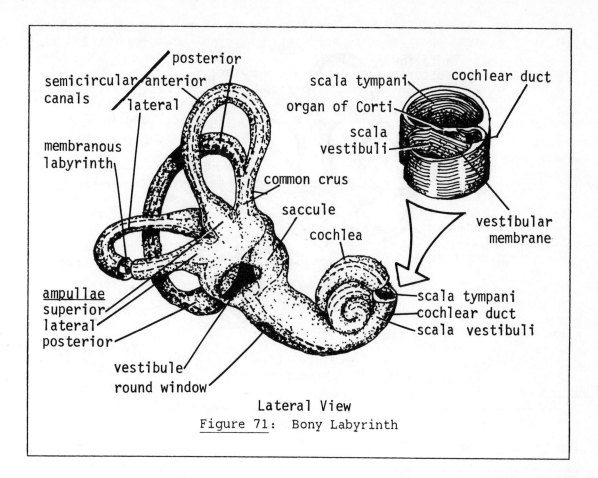

Lateral View
Figure 71:  Bony Labyrinth

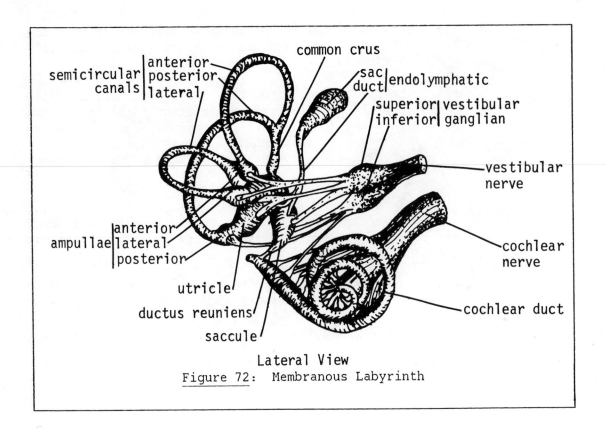

Lateral View

Figure 72:  Membranous Labyrinth

## 6.4 Theories of Hearing

Theories of hearing have been generally grouped into the theory of PLACE and the FREQUENCY theories.  The division between the two theories, however, is not distinct or clear.

1.  The PLACE THEORY  historically has been divided  into two groups: RESONANCE and WAVE theories.

    a.  The resonance theory postulated by  Helmholtz in 1857 considered the cochlea as a series of tuned resonators (vibrators) with the high tones (frequencies) detected at the base of the cochlea and  the low tones detected at the apex.

    b.  The RESONANCE THEORY  was also based on OHM'S  LAW and the DOCTRINE OF SPECIFIC ENERGY OF NERVES.

        i.  OHM'S LAW,  a mathematical theorum by Fourier, stated that any sound wave,  so long as it is periodic,  consists of  the sum  of a  series of  sine waves,  whose frequencies are integral multiples of the fundamental frequency.

      ii.  This means the ear performs an analysis by breaking down the complex sound wave into individual sine wave parts.

     iii.  The DOCTRINE OF SPECIFIC ENERGY OF NERVES stated that the effects produced by stimulation of a nerve are specific to a particular sense organ with which the nerve is associated, i.e. stimulation of optic nerve results in sensation of light, not pressure, etc.

c.  Helmholtz thought the rods of Corti were the vibrating source, but later changed his theory when it was found that nerve fibers do not end on the rods of Corti but rather on hair cells.

d.  Helmholtz revised his theory to account for this discovery and thus began the wave theory or non-resonating theory.

e.  The TRAVELING WAVE theory developed by von Bekesy is not really a traveling wave. This theory states that stimulation of the hair cells along the basilar membrane of the cochlea occurs at the place of greatest amplitude (height) of the pressure wave.

f.  The displacement wave travels from the stapes to the helicotrema.

2.  FREQUENCY THEORIES can be subdivided into two theories: nonanalytic and analytic.

  a.  The NONANALYTIC THEORY is also called the telephone theory.

      i.  This theory supposed that any hair cell from the base to the apex of the cochlea can be stimulated by a sound of any frequency. Therefore, a single cell could give rise to different auditory frequencies.

        1)  Psychological perception of pitch and quality are learned and, therefore, a brain function.

        2)  Opponents of this theory state that single nerve fibers can't fire fast enough to account for the high frequencies that persons detect.

  b.  The ANALYTIC THEORY is illustrated by the Volley Theory.

i.   The VOLLEY THEORY is really a compromise between
     the Place Theory and the Frequency Theory.

ii.  It states that the frequency of sound is determined
     by the nerve cells firing in volleys.

iii. When a single cell reaches its limit of capability,
     an additional nerve begins to respond.

iv.  The two nerves then discharge alternately and are
     capable of doubling the rate or response.

v.   This theory explains frequency response by suppos-
     ing that sound from 15 Hz (cycles per second) to
     400 Hz is based on the frequency of nerve stimula-
     tion (Volley Theory); for frequencies 400 Hz to
     5000 Hz the "place" and "frequency" of excitement
     along the basilar membrane determine the pitch; and
     for frequencies above 5000 Hz pitch is determined
     by nerves firing at the "place" of excitement.

vi.  Loudness is represented by the number of fibers
     active and the rate at which they fire.

## 6.5 Physiological Implications

Neurophysiology of hearing is encompassed in the complex network of the
central auditory nervous system. How this system works is not fully
understood. The practical question still being sought is twofold:

1. How can pressure waves in the cochlea be converted into discrete
   frequency representations of the external stimulus -- including
   its intensity.

2. How does the resultant electrical signal go from the cochlea to
   higher brain centers, with its multitude of connections, and
   still maintain the characteristics of the original signal.

The answer to the first question may, at present, be closer to being
answered. The answer appears to lie in the theories previously discussed. By utilizing the traveling wave and place theory explanation
can be given to why humans are able to detect and discriminate thousands
of frequencies. It has been determined that an individual can detect
1400 pitch changes through the audible frequency ranks and in combination with intensity variation detection abilities is able to distinguish
400,000 intensity/frequency combinations.

Investigations to answer the second question seem to raise more questions about the auditory neural network. What is known, is that an auditory signal maintains its own characteristic throughout the neural pathways. As the signal is transmitted from the lower centers of the brain to higher centers the signal results in a more complex sensation.

It has been speculated that the lower centers of the brain function to analyze the signal for protection. That is, the signal triggers localization responses and may stimulate a reflexive flight response to remove the organism from danger. At the highest centers of the brain (cortex), sounds are associated with more complex human behaviors. There is some evidence that there are specific neural detectors at these higher brain centers that process the distinctive features of language. Recent medical research suggests that there are regions (pathways) of the brain that function to analyze specific parts of speech and that humans may decode speech in association with the movements used to produce speech. Such a model as suggested is called the MOTOR THEORY OF SPEECH PERCEPTION.


## 6.6 Clinical Applications

Disorders of hearing and their symptoms can be differentiated by the location of the problem: outer, middle, and/or inner ear. Conditions that affect the outer and middle ear are referred to as CONDUCTIVE impairments. Inner ear disorders are categorized as SENSORINEURAL impairments.

When there exists a condition in the outer or middle ear that interrupts the normal flow of sound vibration, a conductive hearing loss occurs. Children commonly have a conductive loss accompanying a cold when fluid may accumulate in the middle ear. This infection in the middle ear is called OTITIS MEDIA. There are many forms of otitis media, all of which may prevent the tympanic membrane and ossicular chain from vibrating normally.

In the external auditory meatus wax (cerumen) may accumulate and act as a plug to block the transmission of sound. Audiologists and physicians also report observing blockage of the canal by such objects as pencil erasers, beans, paper, and insects.

Congenital deformities of the outer ear occur as a result of malformation during the embryonic stage. Such conditions as a missing auricle, atresia (closure) of the auditory meatus, or abnormal ossicular chain development may result from branchial arch abnormalities.

Disorders of conduction can be observed by the results of auditory pure-tone testing. As a general rule, individuals with a conductive hearing loss have difficulty with low frequency sounds (125 Hz - 500 Hz). Bone conduction represents the vibration of the bones of the skull (i.e. petrous portion of temporal bone) causing the fluid of the inner ear to vibrate, resulting in the sensation of sound. This audiometric procedure allows the audiologist to by-pass the middle ear and, therefore, assess inner ear function directly. The left panel in Figure 73 shows typical results from a conductive loss test, as seen by the audiogram. The circles (O) indicate the client's threshold (detection) level for pure tone frequency tested in the right ear. The loss of hearing acuity is for the low frequencies. The "arrowhead" (<) symbol represents the client's response level for bone conduction. In this case, the client had bone conduction hearing threshold levels within normal limits. Such an audiogram suggests to the audiologist that the inner ear is functioning normally, and that the loss of hearing is due to the failure of the outer or middle ear to transmit sound appropriately.

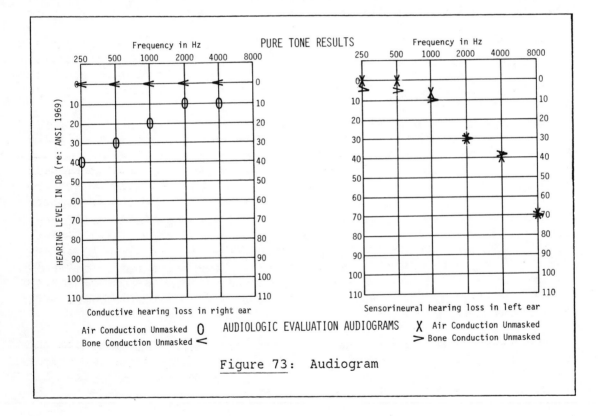

Figure 73: Audiogram

Treatment for a conductive loss generally involved medical treatment to eliminate the source of infection or to remove the blockage. Usually this results in the restoration of normal hearing. Early observation, detection, and intervention are necessary to prevent permanent damage of the middle ear structures.

Sensorineural hearing impairment indicates dysfunction of the inner ear or along the eighth cranial nerve to the brain. The disorder is present when the inner ear cannot analyze the pressure changes of the fluid in the cochlea. Typically this type of loss is marked by normal hearing in the low frequencies and difficulty with sound above 1000 Hz (see right panel of Figure 73).

Congenital inner ear abnormalities may cause a sensorineural hearing loss. This results in congenital deafness. Sensorineural loss may also result from conditions acquired during life, such as trauma to the inner ear from injury, the effects of certain drugs, prolonged exposure to very loud sounds, infections, diseases such as measles, and the effects of aging. An estimated 25 percent of the population have a sensorineural loss by their 70th birthday. By age 80, 50 percent have some loss. This type of loss due to age is called PRESBYCUSIS. Tumors that impinge on the eighth cranial nerve from the cochlea to the brain will result in sensorineural impairment.

Sensorineural losses may or may not be helped by treatment procedures. Medical treatment may arrest further loss but, as yet, restoration of hearing without mechanical help, such as with a hearing aid, is not possible. Hearing aids amplify (increase) the sound presented to the inner ear for analysis.

Unfortunately, not all individuals can benefit from an aid. If the ear is deficient solely in appropriately analyzing the intensity of the incoming message, then by strengthening the signal the individual will benefit. This will help the person to either appropriately detect the signal or provide enough information to assist the person in speech reading (lip reading) so that by visual cues he/she understands the message. For an individual whose hearing deficit causes a severe distortion of the signal, not just an attenuation of the sound, an aid may only result in the amplification of the "noise" and be of little help to the person. However, individuals having sensorineural losses with mild-to-moderate distortion do benefit from the additional auditory cues provided by the hearing aid.

Audiometric testing involves both pure tone (via air conduction and bone conduction) and IMPEDANCE measures. Impedance is the degree a structure opposes forces that are directed against it. Factors that affect impedance are: mechanical friction; the size or mass of the structure; and the compliance (stiffness) of the structure to accommodate forces against it. The combination of these mechanical attributes constitutes the impedance of the hearing structures. IMMITTANCE is now a commonly used term that deals with impedance and its reciprocal, ADMITTANCE.

Impedance testing involves three procedures: tympanometry, static compliance, and acoustic reflex. Tympanometry is a measure of compliance; a test of the mobility of the tympanic membrane. A stiff (noncompliant) ear drum will have the effect of reducing the sound transmission effectiveness of the structure, particularly for low frequencies. The compliance of the tympanic membrane is measured by introducing varying air pressures into the external ear canal.

STATIC COMPLIANCE is a measure of compliance of the middle ear at rest -- without varying pressure changes. Static compliance determines the physical volume plus compliance of the conductive mechanism of the external ear. If the client has a perforation of the tympanic membrane, the volume recording will be larger than expected because measurement will include both the volume of the external canal and the volume of the middle ear space. Normal static compliance values of the external ear vary as a function of age and sex.

ACOUSTIC REFLEX is the measure of normal contraction of the stapedius muscle in both ears when a loud sound (70 to 90 db) is presented to one ear. Normal stapedius reflex has been theorized to be a protective maneuver to protect the hearing structures from damage due to excessively intense sound. When the muscle contracts the ossicular chain stiffens and has a dampening effect on the sound energy. Abnormal acoustic reflex recordings may indicate to the audiologist the possibility of conductive pathology, retrocochlear lesion (cranial nerve VIII pathology), and may serve to provide an estimate of sensorineural impairment.

An audiometric procedure that is receiving increased attention is BRAIN STEM EVOKED RESPONSE (BSER). This procedure assesses the response to sound of the neural system from the cochlea and eighth cranial nerve through the brain stem. As the sound travels through the auditory system nerve impulse activity is recorded by electrodes placed on the client's head. Such specific recordings have been an outgrowth of brain wave activity (electroencephalographic) measurements.

By measuring the appearance or latency of one or a combination of several peaks in the recorded signal the audiologist may make judgment about the presence of cochlea and/or eighth nerve lesion. Evoked potentials (signal peaks) indicate that the auditory neural system has "alerted" the brain's higher centers, but it does not mean the individual can process the information meaningfully. This technique provides an objective assessment of client neural acoustic integrity because it does not rely on the voluntary response of the client which may be subject to bias.

The capacity of the brain to analyze and associate meaning to information transmitted through the peripheral auditory system is referred to as CENTRAL AUDITORY PROCESSING. Central auditory processing disabilities may occur in the absence of peripheral hearing impairment. Distinctive characteristic auditory difficulties associated with both peripheral and central auditory processing dysfunction would include: faulty transmission of the incoming signal; increased sensitivity to noise; reduced attending behavior that may be due to the lack of experience with listening tasks. Specific learning disabilities may be attributed to such central dysfunction.   For example, children who fail or perform poorly on  reading and spelling tasks may suffer  from a central auditory dysfunction.   These  individuals may demonstrate inattentive behavior, sequencing difficulties, problems discriminating auditory input in the presence of distractions  or competing noises in the classroom, play yard, cafeteria, or radio, television,  or conversation background distractors.

Individuals with  a central  auditory processing  dysfunction benefit from specific educational remediation through  a variety of multisensory approaches.   It is important that the child associate visual,  tactual, kinesthetic sensory information with the correct auditory stimulus.   It is also important  to provide the person with  language,  learning,  and social enrichment opportunities which help him  or her to discover areas of strength.

## Glossary

acoustics:    The science of sound, including the production, transmission and effects of mechanical vibrations and waves in any medium, whether audible or not.

air conduction:    The normal passage of sound waves through the ear canal to the drum membrane.

amplitude:    The absolute value to represent the displacement from zero value during one period of the sound wave.

anacusis:    Total deafness.

attenuate:    To reduce in intensity or amount.

audiogram:    A graphic summary of the measurement of hearing level.

audiology:    The study of the entire field of hearing including the anatomy and function of the ear, impairment of hearing, and the educaton or re-education of the person with hearing loss.

aural:    Pertaining to the ear or to the sensation of hearing.  Same as auditory.

ausculation:    The act of listening for sounds within the body.

binaural:    Pertaining to both ears.

bone conduction:    The transmission of sound waves through the head bones to the inner ear.

cerumen:    Wax-like secretion found in the external canal of the ear.

decibel:    A logarithmic ratio unit indicating by what proportion one intensity of sound pressure level differs from another; the decibel is equal to approximately one just noticeable difference in loudness under certain conditions; sometimes inaccurately called a sensation unit.

myringotomy:    Surgical incision of the tympanic membrane.

otitis media:    Inflammation of the middle ear.

otolaryngology:    The single specialty of otology and laryngology.

otology:    The study and treatment of diseases of the ear.

otosclerosis:    The formation of spongy bone in the labyrinth of the ear; especially such growth around the footplate of the stapes impeding its movements in the oval window.

presbycusis:    The diminution of hearing acuity associated with old age.

threshold of hearing:    That level at which sound sensations are first perceived; this is usually accomplished through the use of an audiometer.

vertigo:    A sensation of whirling or dizziness from overstimulation of the semicicular canal receptors; often associated with disease of the ear and deafness.

# References

American Speech, Language, and Hearing Association (1978).  Guidelines for manual pure tone threshold audiometry.  ASHA, 20, 297-301.

American Speech, Language, and Hearing Association (1981).  Prevalence estimates of communication disorders in the U.S.  Language, hearing, and vestibular disorders.  ASHA, 23, 229-237.

Chermak, G. D. (1981).  Handbook of audiological rehabilitation. Springfield, IL: Thomas.

Deutsch, L. G., & Richards, A. M. (1979).  Elementary hearing science. Baltimore:  University Park Press.

Grady, D. (1982).  A sound approach to better hearing.  Discover, 3, 92-99.

Martin, F. N. (1975).  Introduction to audiology.  Englewood Cliffs, NJ: Prentice Hall.

Newby, H. A. (1979).  Audiology (4th ed.).  Englewood Cliffs, NJ: Prentice Hall.

von Bekesy, G. (1957).  The ear.  Scientific American, 8, 2-11.

# Chapter 7
# Nervous System

Earlier chapters have been concerned with the isolated structures of the speech and hearing mechanism.    Now it is necessary to consider the instrument that has the task of setting into motion and coordinating the intricate human machine.  The nervous system is responsible for communication and integration of all bodily functions.   It is a system so complex that it records all experiences,    stores the information for later use,   and is  capable of making instantaneous adjustments  to changes in the environment and using these  changes to facilitate learning.   Individuals are  at times capable  of consciously controlling  their activities, and at other times the system functions without apparent conscious control.  As long as the system is healthy, one gives it little thought; when it breaks down, thought may become difficult.

## 7.1 Divisions of the Nervous System

Central Nervous System

The CENTRAL NERVOUS SYSTEM (CNS) is a functional continuous unit that is divided into the brain and the spinal cord (Figure 74).

1.  The BRAIN lies within the cranial cavity.

2.  The SPINAL  CORD is a  continuous extension  of the brain  and is protected by the vertebral column.

3.  The transition  of the  brain and spinal  cord occurs  through an opening at the base of the cranium known as the MAGNUM FORAMEN.

4.  The CNS has a membrane covering called the MENINGES that consists of three layers.

    a.  The  PIA MATER  is a  transparent  vascular covering  that adheres to the outer surface of the brain and spinal cord.

    b.  The ARACHNOID membrane is the middle layer.

    c.  The DURA  MATER is  the outer membrane  that is  thick and durable and lies  up against the bone  (cranium and vertebrae).

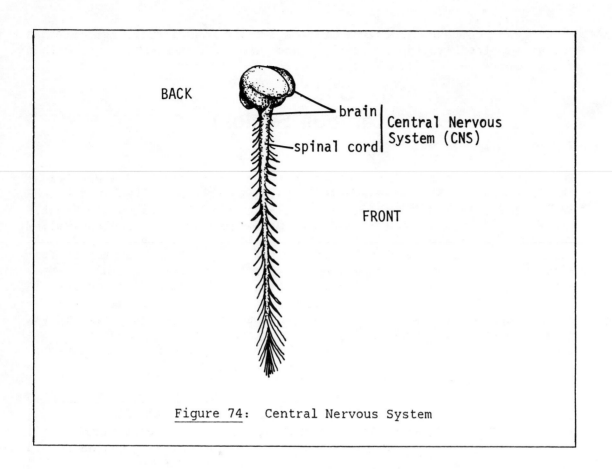

BACK

brain |
          | Central Nervous
spinal cord| System (CNS)

FRONT

Figure 74:  Central Nervous System

## Peripheral Nervous System

The PERIPHERAL NERVOUS SYSTEM (PNS) includes sensory receptors and nerves outside the central nervous system.

1. Twelve pairs of cranial nerves exit from the MIDBRAIN and BRAIN STEM.

2. Thirty-one pairs of spinal nerves exit from the spinal cord and pass through the vertebral column.

## Autonomic Nervous System

The AUTONOMIC NERVOUS SYSTEM controls the "involuntary" activities of the body and include mechanisms of both the CNS and the PNS.

1. This system regulates glands, smooth muscles, and the heart.

2.  Two  components of  the system  are the  SYMPATHETIC system  that
    functions to expend energy,  and  the PARASYMPATHETIC system that
    conserves bodily energy.

## 7.2 Neurons

The NEURON is the basic unit of the nervous system down which electrical
impulses travel.   If the signal is traveling toward the CNS it is sending sensory  information,  and is  called an AFFERENT  signal.   Signals
transmitted  away from  the CNS  are  motor impulses  to muscles  called
EFFERENT signals.

Structure of Neurons

The structure of  the neuron may vary  depending on its location  in the
body.

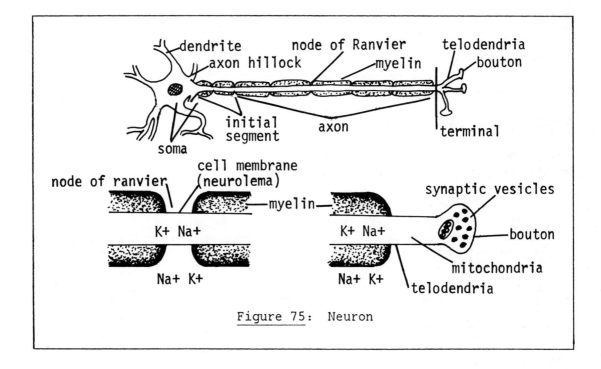

Figure 75:  Neuron

1.  A "typical" neuron has three basic components (Figure 75).

    a.  DENDRITES are projections that receive information.

---

      b.   The CELL  BODY is the  "heart" of  the neuron and  is also capable of receiving information.

      c.   The AXON leaves the cell body  and sends information on to another neuron or end organ.

2.   The type  of neuron  depends on the  number of  processes arising from the cell body.

      a.   A neuron with no dentrites and a single axon is a UNIPOLAR neuron.

      b.   The BIPOLAR neuron is a single  axon and dendrite which is usually sensory.

      c.   The MULTIPOLAR neuron  is a single axon,  many dendrites, and is usually motor.

## Nerve Impulses

Impulses that  travel through the  nerve are  the same whether  they are sending sensory or motor information.   The  stimulus to excite a neuron to generate an impulse may be mechanical, chemical, electrical, or thermal.   To be effective the stimuli must have at least a minimum intensity and duration.

1.   A nervous impulse,  called a spike,  results from a change in the electrochemical difference between the outside  and inside of the cell membrane (Figure 76).

2.   This  change  in  EQUILIBRIUM  (polarization)  results  in DEPOLARIZATION of the cell membrane.

3.   When a stimulus  is so strong it results  in depolarization,  the resultant electrical signal  travels like a wave  over the entire length of the neuron.   This phenomenon is called the ALL OR NONE LAW.

4.   As  the signal  passes  down the neuron,  the cell  immediately attempts to achieve  a neutral state of normal  polarization by a PROCESS OF REPOLARIZATION.   This may be explained by the sodium-potassium PUMP THEORY.   During the readjustment period, the cell is relatively impermeable to another stimulus.

5.   The speed at which an impulse  travels is directly related to the diameter of the nerve axon.

      a.   Propagation is also affected by MYELINIZATION of the axon.

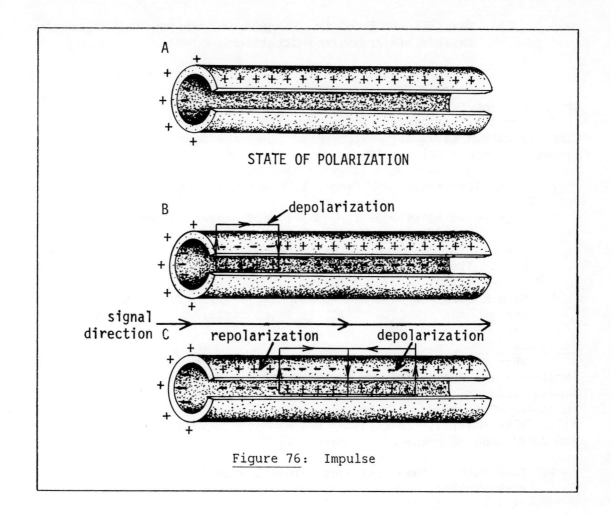

Figure 76:  Impulse

b.  Myelin is  a white fatty  material that covers  some axons and serves as an electrical insulator.

c.  The myelin sheath  is usually found on  the "larger" axons and is found on axons outside  and inside the central nervous system.

d.  The myelin is interrupted at intervals by NODES OF RANVIER which  expose the  axon to  the  outside environment  and, therefore,  may also aid the depolarization process of the axon.

e.  Beneath the myelin and covering all axons is NEURILEMMA.

f.  Neurilemma is found  primarily outside the CNS  and serves in the regeneration of axons that have been injured.

g.  Thus, as a rule of thumb, axons outside the CNS regenerate
while those within the CNS do not.

## Synaptic Transmission of Nerve Impulses

SYNAPTIC TRANSMISSION is the term used when the impulse from one neuron
passes to another (Figure 77).

1.  Endings of axons have finger-like extensions called TELODENDRIA.

2.  Each telodendria ends in a small enlargement called a BOUTON.

3.  The bouton does not actually touch the next dendrite or cell
    body.  It is separated by a SYNAPTIC CLEFT.

4.  Within each bouton are MITOCHONDRIA,  which supply the cell with
    energy, and SYNAPTIC VESICLES, which contain a chemical transmit-
    ter.

5.  When the electrical impulse arrives at the bouton, the mitochond-
    ria are  activated and in turn,  cause the synaptic  vesicles to
    release a chemical (acetylcholine).

6.  This chemical flows into the synaptic  cleft and acts to depolar-
    ize the membrane of the next cell.

7.  The nerve  that  releases  the  chemical  is  known  as  the
    POST-SYNAPTIC NEURON.

8.  The acetylcholine quickly  becomes ineffective,  but while  it is
    active it produces a small depolarization known as the EXCITATORY
    POSTSYNAPTIC POTENTIAL (EPSP).

    a.  If this localizing  effect does not reach  threshold,  the
        nerve impulse ends.

    b.  Or, the effect of subsequent or simultaneous impulses from
        other bouton may increase  the EPSP  so  that the  nerve
        fires.

9.  Impulses from the post-synaptic nerve may have an additive effect
    over time to  stimulate the succeeding neurons.   This effect is
    called TEMPORAL SUMMATION.

10. Also, boutons from one or more axons  may act upon a single den-
    drite or cell body to continue the impulse through the succeeding
    neuron.  This effect is SPACIAL SUMMATION.

11. Synaptic Transmission may be either EXCITATORY or INHIBITORY.

a.  The excitatory synapse, as previously discussed, results in depolarization (EPSP) of the presynaptic membrane.

b.  The inhibitory synapse produces an opposite effect by hyperpolarizing the presynaptic membrane, and thus preventing the impulse being transmitted. This is called INHIBITORY POSTSYNAPTIC POTENTIAL (IPSP).

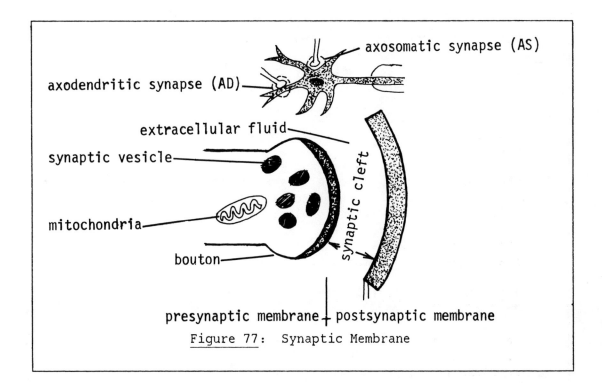

Figure 77:  Synaptic Membrane

## 7.3 Divisions of the Central Nervous System

Brain and Spinal Cord

Deriving from the neural tube (and not losing its hollow aspect) the CNS has developed numerous divisions (Figure 78).

1.  The PROSENCEPHALON (forebrain) is subdivided into two subdivisions.

    a.  The TELENCEPHALON has as its primary derivation the CEREBRAL CORTEX.

    b.  The DIENCEPHALON includes the THALAMUS.

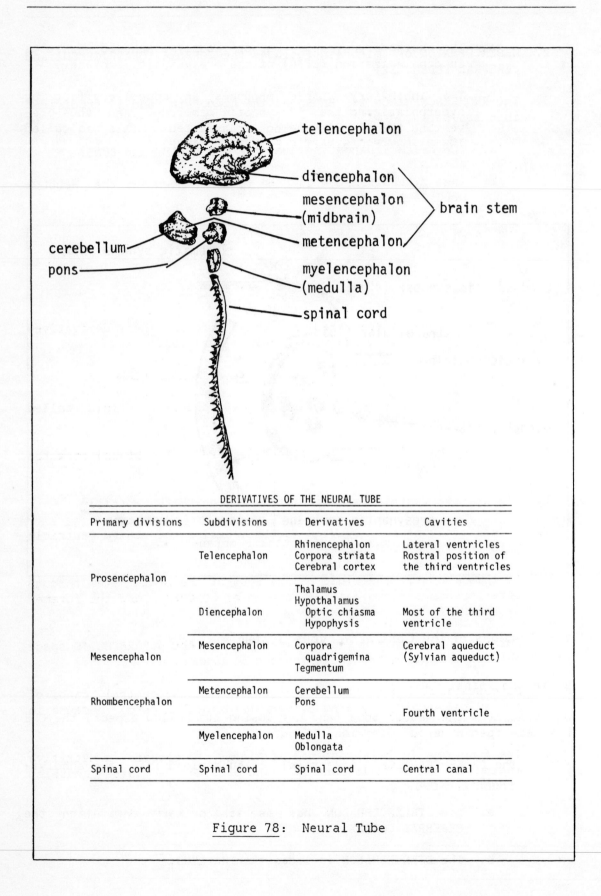

DERIVATIVES OF THE NEURAL TUBE

| Primary divisions | Subdivisions | Derivatives | Cavities |
|---|---|---|---|
| Prosencephalon | Telencephalon | Rhinencephalon<br>Corpora striata<br>Cerebral cortex | Lateral ventricles<br>Rostral position of<br>the third ventricles |
| | Diencephalon | Thalamus<br>Hypothalamus<br>  Optic chiasma<br>  Hypophysis | Most of the third<br>ventricle |
| Mesencephalon | Mesencephalon | Corpora<br>  quadrigemina<br>Tegmentum | Cerebral aqueduct<br>(Sylvian aqueduct) |
| Rhombencephalon | Metencephalon | Cerebellum<br>Pons | Fourth ventricle |
| | Myelencephalon | Medulla<br>Oblongata | |
| Spinal cord | Spinal cord | Spinal cord | Central canal |

Figure 78:  Neural Tube

2.  MESENCEPHALON or midbrain includes the CORPORA QUADRIGEMENI and CEREBRAL PEDUNCLES.

3.  The RHOMBENCEPHALON is known as the hindbrain and is subdivided into two parts.

    a.  The METENCEPHALON includes the CEREBELLUM and PONS.

    b.  The MYELENCEPHALON is the region known as the MEDULLA OBLONGATA.

4.  The final division is the SPINAL CORD.


## Ventricles

The primary divisions of the brain and spinal cord and their derivatives surround four cavities known as ventricles (Figure 79).

1.  The ventricles contain structures called CHOROID PLEXUS.

2.  The choroid plexus manufacture a colorless fluid called CEREBROSPINAL FLUID.

3.  Two large cavities (one in each hemisphere of the brain) form the LATERAL ventricles.

4.  The lateral ventricles drain into a common THIRD ventricle.

5.  A relatively narrow SYLVIAN AQUEDUCT drains the third ventricle into the FOURTH ventricle.

6.  At this point, the fluid passes out of the brain stem through three openings: two lateral foramen of LUSCHKA; and the foramen of MAGENDIE.

7.  Outside the brain the fluid circulates in the SUBARACHNOID space between the pia mater and arachnoid membranes.

8.  Cerebrospinal fluid does not circulate in the central canal of the spinal cord (only around the outside of the cord) because in humans the canal is usually closed off.

9.  The function of cerebrospinal fluid is to provide a nutritive medium to nerve cells and it also provides a "water" cushion around the CNS.

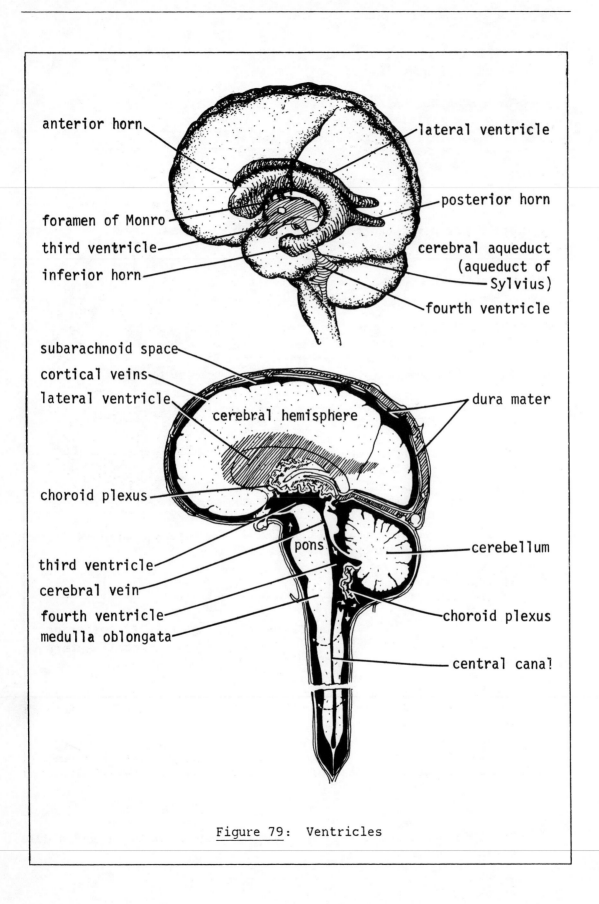

Figure 79:  Ventricles

## 7.4 Blood Supply

BLOOD to the brain is supplied by two pairs of arteries (Figure 80).

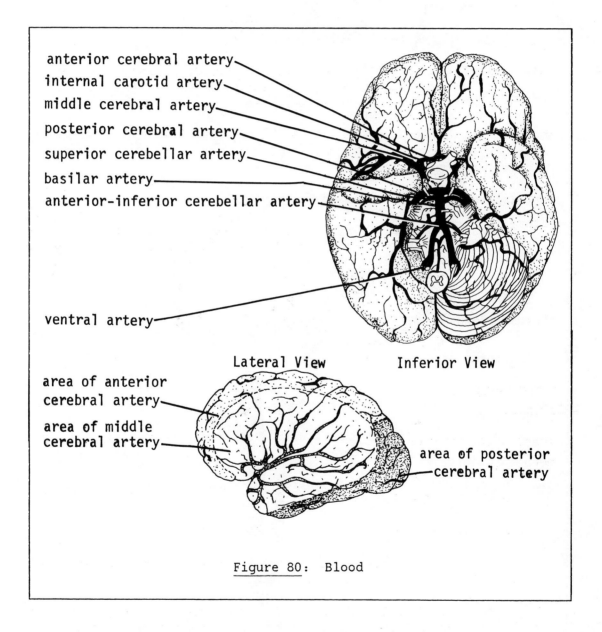

anterior cerebral artery

internal carotid artery

middle cerebral artery

posterior cerebral artery

superior cerebellar artery

basilar artery

anterior-inferior cerebellar artery

ventral artery

Lateral View          Inferior View

area of anterior
cerebral artery

area of middle
cerebral artery

area of posterior
cerebral artery

Figure 80:  Blood

1.  The INTERNAL CAROTID arteries divide  into an anterior and middle
    cerebral artery.

a. The ANTERIOR CEREBRAL ARTERY supplies the longitudinal "midline" area of the cerebral hemisphere.

b. The MIDDLE CEREBRAL ARTERY is the largest branch and serves the lateral surface of the cerebrum.

2. The VERTEBRAL artery becomes known as the BASILAR ARTERY at the level of the pons and POSTERIOR CEREBRAL ARTERY when it reaches the cerebrum.

a. The basilar artery ascends in front of the brain stem.

b. The posterior cerebral artery supplies the lower part of the lateral cerebrum (temporal area) and the posterior visual region (occipital area).

3. A ring of blood vessels (arterial circle) at the base of the brain is formed by the union of the anterior cerebral arteries and the posterior cerebral arteries.

a. This ring is called the CIRCLE OF WILLIS.

b. The Circle of Willis functions to equalize circulation of blood in the brain and assures that, in the case of damage to one artery, blood will reach the brain through other avenues.

## 7.5 Structures of the Brain

Cerebrum

The CEREBRUM is the largest part of the human brain and is the outer covering that typically is represented as the "brain" (Figure 81).

1. The appearance is characterized as "gray" (composed largely of bodies of nerve cells).

2. There are numerous convolutions called GYRI.

3. The irregular grooves or invaginations are called either FISSURES or SULCI.

a. The LONGITUDINAL FISSURE is a large fissure which gives the appearance of dividing the cerebrum into two cerebral hemispheres. The hemispheres are actually connected deep by fibers of the CORPUS CALLOSUM.

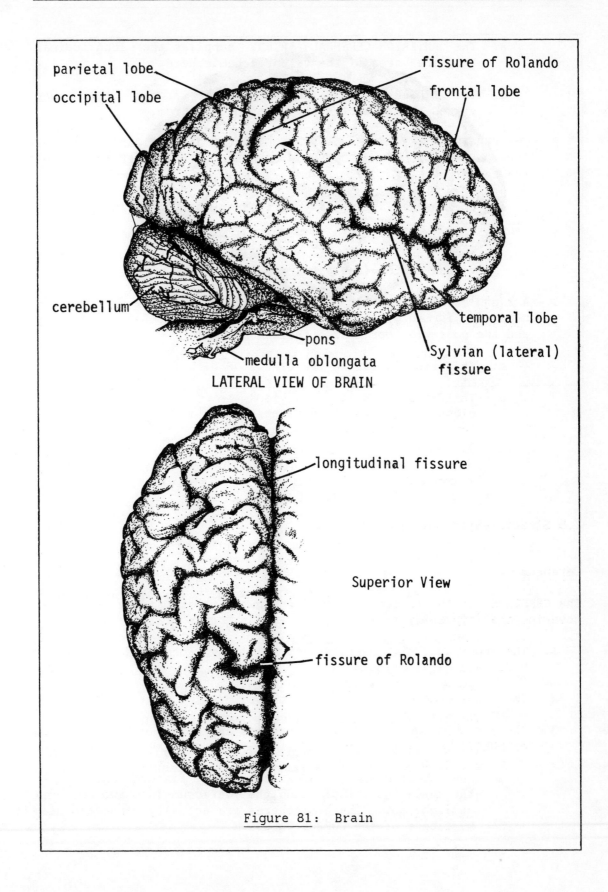

Figure 81:  Brain

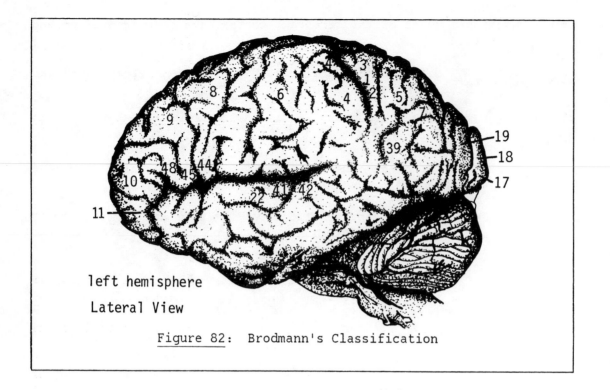

left hemisphere

Lateral View

Figure 82:   Brodmann's Classification

b.  The Sylvian fissure is also known as the "lateral" fissure, and roughly, divides the cerebrum into top and bottom sections.   Specifically, it divides the FRONTAL lobe from the TEMPORAL lobe.

c.  The "central" fissure called the fissure of ROLANDO divides the cerebrum into front and back sections--FRONTAL lobe from the PARIETAL lobe.

4.  The fissures divide each hemisphere into five sections or lobes.

a.  The FRONTAL lobe lies in front of the fissure of Rolando and above the Sylvian fissure.

b.  The PARIETAL lobe lies behind fissure of Rolando and above the posterior half of the Sylvian fissure.

c.  The TEMPORAL lobe is below the Sylvian fissure.

d.  The OCCIPITAL lobe is posterior to the parietal and temporal lobes, behind a parieto-occipital fissure.

e.  The INSULA, also known as the "ISLAND of REIL" lies within the Sylvian fissure.

5.  Functional areas of the cerebral  cortex have been identified and classified.

    a.  To differentiate cellularly distinctive areas CORTICAL MAPS have been devised.

    b.  The most widely used system,  devised by Brodmann,  has 47 areas (Figure 82).

    c.  The Brodmann numerical system differentiates specific areas within three principal areas.

        i.  The motor functions  of the body are  controlled by the large region in front of the fissure of Rolando (precentral cortex).

            1) Area 4 is the  primary motor area responsible for fine volitional movements.

            2) Area 6  is responsible for the  activities of groups of muscles.

        ii.  The SENSORY area of the cortex functions to receive conscious sensory information.

            1) The primary  tactile sensation areas  for the body are located  in Brodmann's Areas  1-3 (post-central fissure).

            2) Visual information is processed  in the occipital lobe with the primary area being 17.

            3) The primary auditory area  is in the temporal lobe Area 41.

        iii.  Association areas of the brain  connect with  the various motor and sensory areas.

            1) It is the tissue  which surrounds the primary areas and is responsible for recall, memory, and accurate differentiation.

            2) Important association areas  for speech  and hearing are  Wernicke's Area  (22),  Broca's Area (44), the ANGULAR GYRUS (39),  and supplementary motor area.

6.  CEREBRAL DOMINANCE is a term used to indicate that certain neural functions  are controlled  primarily  by one hemisphere  of  the brain.

a. Motor functions for movement of the arms, hands, legs, etc. are controlled by the cerebral hemisphere on the opposite side of the body (contralateral representation).

b. The preferential use of one hand or leg over the other is called LATERALITY.

c. Midline structures such as those necessary to maintain life are controlled by both hemispheres.

d. There is also information sent to the brain from the face, for example, which remains on the same side. It has IPSILATERAL representation.

7. The cerebrum is interconnected by fibers (nerves) that are generally three types:

a. ASSOCIATION fibers connect various areas within the cerebral hemispheres.

b. COMMISSURAL fibers connect the two hemispheres. The CORPUS CALLOSUM is the largest group of fibers.

c. PROJECTION fibers connect the cerebrum to lower centers of the central nervous system. These are either afferent (corticopetal) or efferent (corticofugal).

8. The function of the cerebrum is to process all conscious sensations and mediate voluntary movement.


## Diencephalon and Basal Ganglia

Deep to the cerebrum lie two intricate structures known as the diencephalon and basal ganglia (Figure 83).

1. The DIENCEPHALON is a region that includes the thalamus, the optic tracks, and the pituitary body.

a. The THALAMUS is known as the "great relay station" because of its multiple connections with the cerebrum above it and the spinal cord below.

b. The diencephelon plays an important role in the autonomic responses of the body.

2. The BASAL GANGLIA includes such internal areas as the caudate nucleus, globus pallidus, the putamen, claustrum, and amygdala.

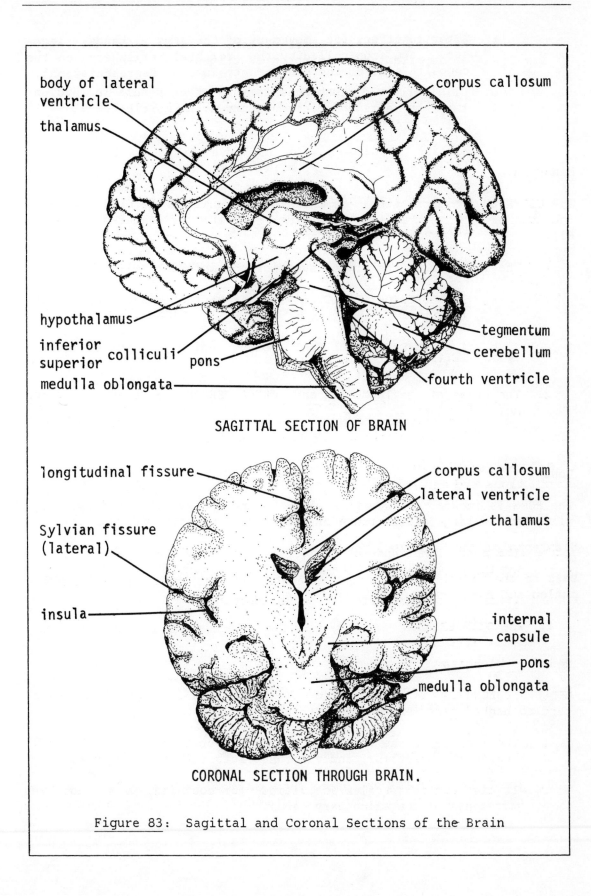

SAGITTAL SECTION OF BRAIN

body of lateral ventricle

thalamus

corpus callosum

hypothalamus

inferior
superior colliculi

pons

medulla oblongata

tegmentum

cerebellum

fourth ventricle

CORONAL SECTION THROUGH BRAIN.

longitudinal fissure

Sylvian fissure
(lateral)

insula

corpus callosum

lateral ventricle

thalamus

internal
capsule

pons

medulla oblongata

Figure 83:  Sagittal and Coronal Sections of the Brain

a.  Mediated by the cerebral cortex,  the basal ganglia plays
    an important role in motor functions.

b.  Clinically,  disturbances to this  area result in involun-
    tary movements and disorders involving muscle tone.

## Midbrain

The MIDBRAIN (mesencephalon)  is the smallest unit of the brain stem and
consists of the  tectum,  the tegmentum,  and the  crura cerebri (Figure
83).

1.  The TECTUM consists of the superior and inferior colliculi.

    a.  The SUPERIOR COLLICULI  is an important visual  relay sys-
        tem.

    b.  The  INFERIOR COLLICULI  relays auditory  impulses to  the
        thalamus.

2.  The areas of the TEGMENTUM and  CRURA CEREBRI serve primarily for
    motor functions.

## Pons

The PONS is located  between the midbrain and the medulla  and is recog-
nized by the large protuberance of the ventral portion. (Figure 83).

1.  The pons  functions to  project fibers  to various  parts of  the
    brain, primarily with the cerebellum and medulla.

2.  It is one of the parts of the "hindbrain".

## Medulla Oblongata

MEDULLA OBLONGATA  is also part  of the  hindbrain and joins  the spinal
cord to higher parts of the brain (Figure 83).

1.  The medulla is the vital center  of the brain because it controls
    heartbeat, breathing, and vasoconstrictors (blood pressure).

2.  It also controls reflex activities  for coughing,  vomiting,  and
    movements of the alimentary canal.

Cerebellum

The CEREBELLUM is the second largest part of the brain and its structure resembles the cerebral hemispheres (Figure 84).

1.  It is divided into two hemispheres by a midline portion, the VERMIS.

2.  For descriptive purposes the cerebellum is divided into four parts.

    a.  The VENTRAL portion receives information about equilibrium.  The ANTERIOR portion and the POSTERIOR portion receive sensory information from the spinal cord.

    b.  The DORSAL portion has extensive connections with the pons and medulla

3.  The principal functions of the cerebellum are threefold.

    a.  It maintains muscle tone

    b.  It serves to coordinate muscle movement.

    c.  It aids the body in the maintenance of equilibrium.

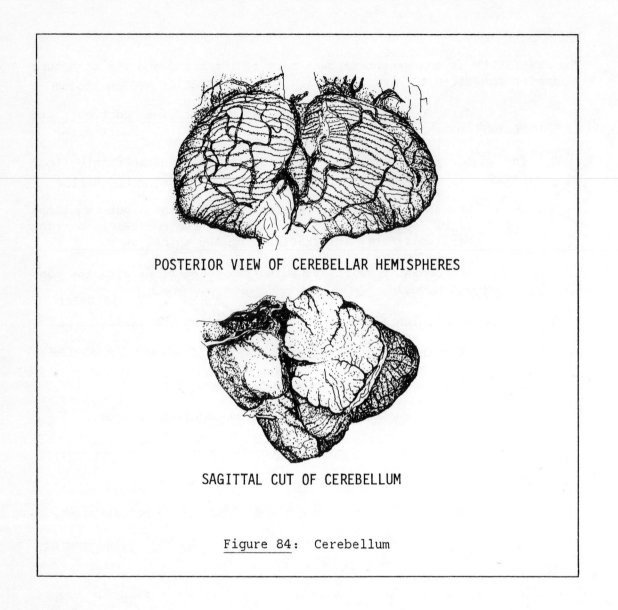

POSTERIOR VIEW OF CEREBELLAR HEMISPHERES

SAGITTAL CUT OF CEREBELLUM

Figure 84:  Cerebellum

## 7.6 Spinal Cord

Structure of the Spinal Cord

The SPINAL CORD extends  from the foramen magnum to the  first or second lumbr vertebrae (Figure 85).

1.  A cross section of the spinal cord reveals a core of gray matter, roughly shaped like the letter "H".

   a.  A narrow midline strip that  connects the two lateral columns is called the GRAY COMMISSURE.

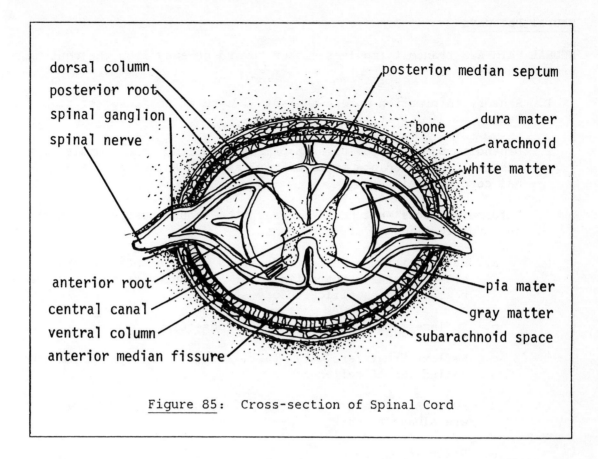

dorsal column
posterior root
spinal ganglion
spinal nerve

posterior median septum

bone
dura mater
arachnoid
white matter

anterior root
central canal
ventral column
anterior median fissure

pia mater
gray matter
subarachnoid space

Figure 85:   Cross-section of Spinal Cord

     b.   The dorsal or posterior columns are called DORSAL HORNS.

     c.   Ventral or anterior columns are commonly called VENTRAL HORNS.

2.   The GRAY MATTER contains cell bodies and is where synapses occur.

3.   WHITE MATTER surrounds the gray matter and is composed of groups of nerve tracts that have similar functions.

     a.   The individual tracts are sometimes referred to as FASCICULI.

     b.   The fasciculi are grouped into three FUNICULI which divide the white matter.

4.   The dorsal, lateral, and ventral areas of white matter contain descending and ascending pathways.

     a.   The descending neuronal fibers convey motor information.

     b.   The ascending convey sensory information.

Neural Pathways

NEURAL PATHWAYS transmit impulses either toward or away from the central nervous system.

1.  Sensory information enters the spinal cord at the level of stimulation.

2.  Depending on the type of sensory stimulation, the impulse may result in an immediate motor REFLEX response anywhere in the spinal cord or brain stem.

3.  Information does not have to reach the conscious level at the cerebrum to elicit a motor response.

    a.  By definition a reflex refers to an involuntary response, either muscle contractions or glandular sensation, in response to specific sensory stimuli.

    b.  Reflexes are predictable and purposeful.

    c.  Reflexes that are very fast, such as an eye blink are called PHASIC reflexes.

    d.  POSTURAL reflexes are longer lasting sustained acts that are always at work.

    e.  Reflexes may be classified in several ways:

        i.  One way is according to the STIMULI that elicit the response.

        ii.  A second way is according to the response that results.

        iii.  Another way is according to the level or complexity of the synapses in the CNS.

        iv.  Finally, they may be classified according to whether the reflex was present at birth or was a learned response.

    f.  The simplest reflex arc consists of an afferent neuron synapsing with an efferent neuron in the same segment of the spinal cord.

    g.  Reflexes may also have a third neuron, INTERNUNCIAL NEURON, that serves as an intermedite neuron between the afferent and efferent impulses.

h.  Intersegmental reflex arcs have their afferent neuron divide into ascending and descending branches that allow a synapse to occur at different segmental levels of the spinal cord.

4.  Spinal reflexes call forth two basic responses.

a.  FLEXION is any response in which the limb bends toward the body and away from the ground.

i.  How much flexion occurs depends on the type of sensory stimulus and the intensity of the stimulus.

ii.  Pain brings forth the greatest flexion response.

b.  EXTENSION response occurs when the limb straightens as in supporting the body against the pull of gravity.

i.  A STRETCH reflex (myotatic reflex) occurs when there is an increase in tension or stretching of a muscle.  This causes the muscle that is stretched to contract.

ii.  This principle is important to muscle groups as well.  When a limb is flexed this creates stretching of the antagonistic muscles (extensors).  The stretching stimulus calls forth a myotatic reflex which makes the extensors contract.

5.  Intersegmental reflexes are different from segmental reflexes only to the extent that the reflexes have a different level of neural organization.

a.  Intersegmental patterns involve greater COOPERATION as well as COMPETITION between reflexes.

b.  Cooperative reflexes aid each other so that a smooth movement is produced.

i.  It is the alternative responses of two reflexes (flexion and extension) that allows a rhythmical pattern.

ii.  The "scratching" of its ear by a dog is a cooperative act and demonstrates RECIPROCAL INHIBITION.

iii.  Simply stated, the reciprocal inhibition is created by a flexor reflex suppressing (inhibiting) an extension response and then the resulting stretching of the extensor muscles set up an extension reflex that suppresses flexion.

c.   Competition reflexes  occur when  several sensory  stimuli
     compete for the motor response.

d.   To determine which reflex "wins", the body has set priori-
     ties for reflexes.

     i.   FLEXION usually ranks first because it is a protec-
          tive device.

     ii.  Next comes the  stronger,  more INTENSE  stimulus
          responses.

     iii. When a reflex has been  operating for sometime,  it
          will lose out to a reflex more recently initiated.

6.  Suprasegmental reflexes  involve control  of either  segmental or
    intersegmental reflexes by the brain.   Generally, these reflexes
    are for postural patterns.


## Neuromuscular Response System

The NEUROMUSCULAR response  system is important to  understanding reflex
activity as well as for volitional movement (Figure 86).

1.  The motor  system for reflexes  and coordination  include various
    structures of the brain and  spinal cord,  nerve structures,  and
    muscles.

    a.   Muscle fibers  are served by  both sensory and  motor neu-
         rons.

    b.   Cell bodies of  the motor neurons are located  in the ven-
         tral horns of the spinal cord.

    c.   From the  ventral horn,  axons  carry the impulses  to the
         muscle and end in FIBRILS (footplates) upon muscle fibers.

         i.   Each axon divides into a number of footplates but a
              muscle fiber has only one axon fibril.

         ii.  Therefore, one motor neuron has complete control of
              a number of muscle fibers.

2.  There are two kinds of motor innervation of a muscle.

    a.   ALPHA INNERVATION composes the greatest percent  of motor
         fibers innervating  muscles and  functions by  causing the
         muscles to contract.

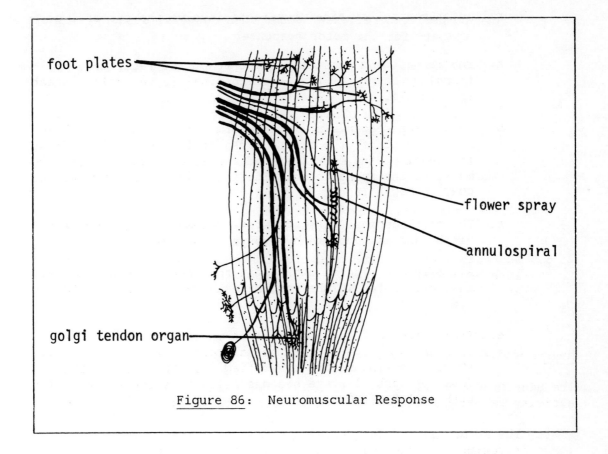

foot plates

flower spray

annulospiral

golgi tendon organ

Figure 86:  Neuromuscular Response

b.  The GAMMA EFFERENT  are specialized motor fibers  that act
to affect the sensitivity of muscle receptors.

   i.  The principal  receptor is called a  MUSCLE SPINDLE
that records the "stretch" of a muscle fiber.

  ii.  There are two specialized muscle spindle receptors:
annulospiral endings and flowerspray endings.

iii.  A second type of receptor is the GOLGI TENDON organ
that records tension within  the muscle tendon system.

  iv.  The  job of gamma efferent  is  to affect sensory
information returning from the  muscle,  and therefore allow  a feedback system that  regulates vital
information  about  the  functioning  of the  muscle
fiber.   This is important  to kinesthetic information.

3. Neural motor control of fine  movements involve the cerebral cortex.

   a. The largest and  most important tract to  facilitate voli-
      tional movement  is the  corticospinal (pyramidal)  tract
      (Figure 87).

   b. This tract descends primarily form  Area 4 (giant cells of
      Betz);  most of  the fibers cross to the  opposite side at
      the level of the medulla,  and course down to various seg-
      ments of the spinal cord.  The tract is called the LATERAL
      CORTICOSPINAL TRACT.

   c. The corticospinal  tract system  becomes myelinated  after
      birth, and is complete by two years of age.

   d. All efferent tracts, other than the cortico-spinal system,
      that originate  in the cortex  make up  the EXTRAPYRAMIDAL
      system.

   e. It is important to remember that motor pathways synapse in
      the ventral  horn of the  spinal cord.   The motor neurons
      above this synapse are classified  as UPPER MOTOR NEURONS.
      Those peripheral nerve neurons below this level are called
      LOWER MOTOR NEURONS.

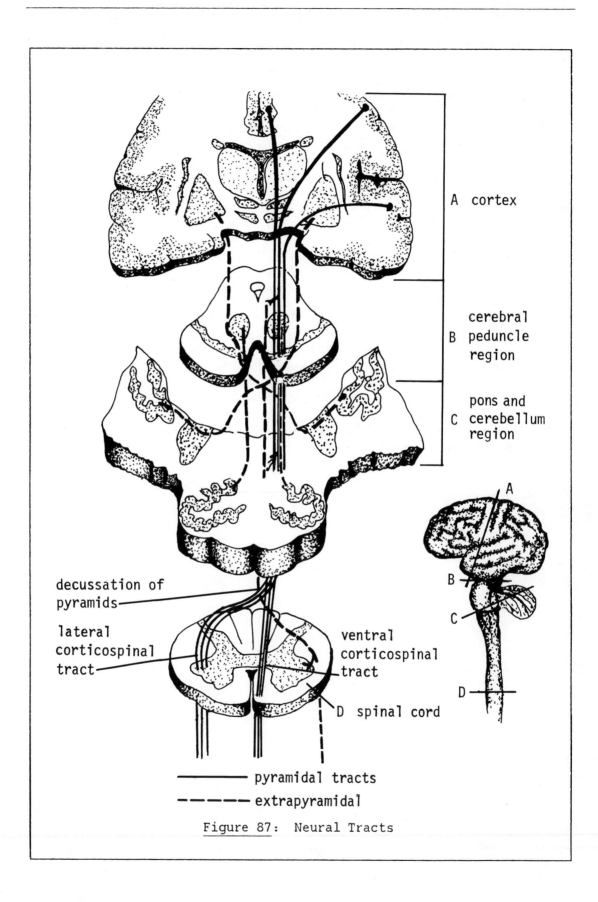

decussation of
pyramids

lateral
corticospinal
tract

ventral
corticospinal
tract

D spinal cord

A cortex

cerebral
B peduncle
region

pons and
C cerebellum
region

————— pyramidal tracts
— — — — extrapyramidal

Figure 87:  Neural Tracts

## 7.7 Cranial Nerves

CRANIAL NERVES are part of the peripheral nervous system that exits from the brain (Figure 88).

1. Three cranial nerves only transmit SENSORY information to the brain.

2. Five of the nerves convey only MOTOR information from the brain.

3. Four cranial nerves have both sensory and motor functions.

4. The twelve pair of cranial nerves have nuclei along the brain stem.

   a. Cranial nerves 1 through 4 are located in the midbrain.

   b. Cranial nerves 5 through 8 lie in the pons.

   c. Cranial nerves 9 through 12 are in the medulla.

5. With the exception of cranial nerve 4, the nerves enter and exit on the same side as they serve.

| NERVE NUMBER | NAME | MOTOR/SENSORY COMPONENTS | FUNCTION |
|---|---|---|---|
| 1 | OLFACTORY | sensory | smell |
| 2 | OPTIC | sensory | vision |
| 3 | OCULOMOTOR | motor | all eye muscles, except lateral rectus and superior oblique |
| 4 | TROCHLEAR | motor | superior oblique (rotates eyeball outward and downward) |
| 5 | TRIGEMINAL | sensory | face, sinuses, teeth |
|  |  | motor | muscles of mastication, hearing (tensor tampini) |
| 6 | ABDUCENS | motor | external rectus (rotates eyeball outward) |
| 7 | FACIAL | sensory | anterior 2/3 of tongue, velum |
|  |  | motor | muscles of face, hearing (stapedius) |
| 8 | ACOUSTIC |  |  |
|  | a. vestibular branch | sensory | maintenance of equilibrium |
|  | b. cochlear or auditory branch | sensory | hearing |
| 9 | GLOSSOPHARYNGEAL | sensory | posterior part of tongue, tonsil, pharynx |
|  |  | motor | pharyngeal musculature |
| 10 | VAGUS | sensory | heart, lungs, trachea, larynx, pharynx, G.I. tract, external ear |
|  |  | motor | lungs, bronchi, G.I. tract |
| 11 | SPINAL ACCESSORY |  |  |
|  | a. cranial portion | motor | pharynx, upper larynx, uvula, palate |
|  | b. spinal portion | motor | upper portion of sternomastoid and trapezius muscles |
| 12 | HYPOGLOSSAL | motor | tongue muscles, strap muscles |

Figure 88:  Cranial Nerves

## 7.8 Spinal Nerves

1.  Thirty-one pairs of SPINAL NERVES exit from the spinal cord, and emerge through intervertebral foramina.

2.  The spinal nerves take their name from the vertebral segments from which they emerge, with these exceptions:

    a.  Cervical nerves 1-7 exit above their corresponding verte-brae.

    b.  Cervical nerve 8 exits below vertebra 7.

3.  Because the spinal cord ends at the top of the lumber segment, spinal nerves from L2-S5 continue down and exit by their corresponding vertebrae.

## 7.9 Clinical Applications

This chapter began by stating that the nervous system was a complex integrated network that controlled our total being. The more one begins to understand the system the more questions are asked. New, high technological advances have allowed in-depth study of motor-sensory innervations. Humans are not necessarily "preprogrammed" to exist in the environment. They are capable, however, of instantaneous adjustments created by their changing environment. From these adaptive maneuvers they "learn" so that the next movement requires less time to execute.

Clinically, motor behaviors have been dichotomized as either voluntary or involuntary. Such classification may now be regarded as an oversimplification. The neural motor system is an interrelated multi-loop-within-loop circuit. Even at the reflexive level it is hypothesized that sensory tracts are capable of memory. That is, at a basic neural level, information may be stored to allow a response to be carried out with less sensory feedback than was originally required.

This complex system allows an individual to make small adjustments in the speech apparatus. Stated another way, this reflex sensorimotor control allows one to execute linguistic rules motorically in a rapid "unthinking" manner, while at the same time he/she is engaged in some other motoric activity.

## Cerebellum and Basal Ganglia

The central and peripheral neural systems are organized and orchestrated in a manner that  allows site of lesion to be  determined by observation of motoric abilities.   Lesions to the cerebellar and  basal ganglia of the brain result in distinctive motor problems.

When there is irregularity of movements while attempting to execute a voluntary act, a cerebellar lesion is suspected.   The role of the cerebellum is to coordinate impulses from  the cerebral cortex during voluntary activity.   A disorder involving  this region results  in impulses improperly  discharged,  and  muscle contractions  are not  coordinated. This type of disorder is known as INTENTION TREMOR.

The cerebellum  is also responsible  for maintaining  bodily posture. It does  so by controlling  afferent (sensory)  information originating from muscle spindles.  The stretch reflexes are inhibited and posture is maintained.   When a lesion prevents the cerebellum from receiving these impulses, the contractions of the muscles are not checked.  For an individual  with this  disorder,  attempting  to  walk or  reach results  in incoordination that is known as ATAXIA.

Lesions to  the BASAL GANGLIA  are characterized by  involuntary contractions,  particularly to the digital and cranial muscles.   The basal ganglia acts to  inhibit certain functions of the  cerebral cortex.   If the lesion is to the  corticospinal (pyramidal)  tract,  the involuntary movements are rapid and jerky.   It  represents a disorder that fails to inhibit spontaneous pyramidal discharge.  These involuntary tremors tend to smooth  out during  voluntary activity or  sleep and therefore,  are known as TREMORS AT REST.   When the extrapyramidal tract is involved, a greater number of muscles of the  body are affected.   This condition is known as CHOREA.   Another result of  basal ganglia defects are abnormal movements of a slow rate,  characterized by a snake-like twisting of the extremities and digital muscles.  This condition is called ATHETOSIS.

## Upper Motor Lesion

Lesions of  the cerebral  cortex generally result  in sensory  and motor defects affecting  the opposite side of  the body.  Involvement  of the cortical motor  areas and motor  cells in  the spinal cord  are commonly referred to as UPPER MOTOR LESIONS.  Therefore, lesions in Area 4 of the cortex and to  the corticospinal tract at the medulla  level are characterized by PARESIS (weakness) on  the CONTRALATERAL (opposite)  side of the body,  involving muscles  concerned with  fine-skilled,  volitional movement.   There is no paralysis because movements to groups of muscles can still be  innervated by the extrapyramidal  system.   Movements lack the facility of  an intact system because Area 6  and the extrapyramidal system does not limit its control to any one muscle.

The most  common and pronounced effect  of upper motor  lesions occur
when both the  pyramidal and extrapyramidal systems  are affected.   One
loses the innervation to individual muscles (pyramidal)  as well as muscle groups (extrapyramidal).   In this  case,  "paralysis" will occur to
varying degrees, depending on the number of tracts involved.  As a rule,
the closer the  lesion to the spinal  cord the chances are  greater that
more tracts will be involved.  Only those biological functions necessary
to sustain life located near midline, and consequently,  the same organs
producing speech, may remain relatively intact,  if the lesion is to one
side only, because of BILATERAL neural control to these areas.

It is  the effect  of the  extrapyramidal tract  lesion that  has the
greatest effect on the body.   The extrapyramidal innervation is capable
of both facilitation as well as  inhibition.   The pyramidal system is
facilitory only.   As the body functions to maintain its posture against
the pull of  gravity stretch reflexes are  continually occurring.   However,  control of these reflexes is impossible and they operate unabated
because there  is no longer  inhibition from the  extrapyramidal system.
The result  is a muscle state  of spasticity,  hypertonus,  and lowered
threshold of these reflexes.

## Dysarthria

A group of  speech disorders characterized by the loss  of muscular control (most commonly reflecting neurological integrity) is referred to as
dysarthria.   The general bodily manifestations of upper motor and cerebellar lesions  that have been  described similarly affected  the speech
process (respiration, articulation, phonation, resonation, and prosody).
The reader should return to chapter  three,  section 3.7,  to review the
disorders that reflect such motor disabilities.

## Lower Motor Lesions

Lesions which occur  in the  ventral root  of  the spinal  cord or  the
peripheral spinal  nerves are termed  lower motor neuron  lesions.   The
consequence of such lesions present  different clinical signs than upper
motor  neuron  lesions  and  result in  ipsilateral motor  and  sensory
defects.   The specific  characteristics when several dorsal  or ventral
roots are severed are that motor  reflexes become impossible because the
reflex arc cannot be completed.   In lesion to the ventral root,  voluntary control to muscles is completely lost.   Muscles deprived of innervation become flaccid (limp)  and  atrophy.   This clinical condition is
termed FLACCID PARALYSIS.

A  different  clinical  condition  exists when  the  dorsal  root  is
involved.   The reflex arc to specific  muscles is lost but paralysis is
not  present because  the  intact ventral  root  still relays  voluntary
information to the muscles.

## Language

Two regions of the cerebral cortex are traditionally discused in speech-language processing:  Area 41 known as WERNICKE'S area;  and Area 44, called BROCA'S area.    These areas are important to speech reception and expression,  but of course,  all regions of the brain play an important role in language.   In general,  speech and language are controlled by the  left hemisphere in  right-handed humans.   The  right hemisphere also plays a role  in language but the extent is  not as clearly defined as with the left hemisphere.  The role each hemisphere plays is shown in (Figure 89).  The cerebral hemispheres are specialized to carry out different cognitive functions  independent of each other.    The left hemisphere assumes the responsibility for  verbal and analytic thought,  and the right hemisphere functions primarily for intuitive processes.   However, the hemispheres are able to cross-reference some functions by communication through the corpus callosum.

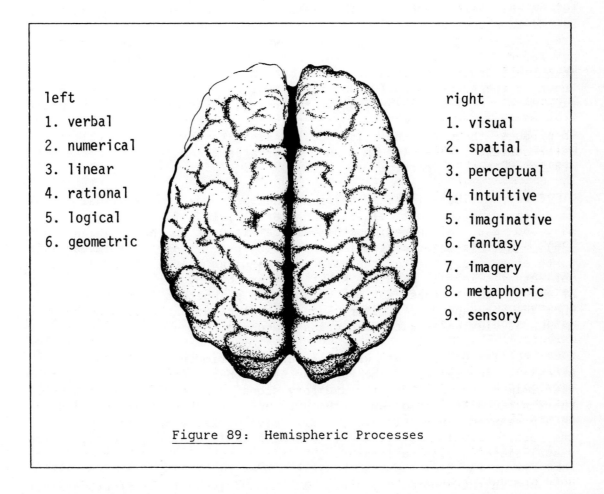

left
1. verbal
2. numerical
3. linear
4. rational
5. logical
6. geometric

right
1. visual
2. spatial
3. perceptual
4. intuitive
5. imaginative
6. fantasy
7. imagery
8. metaphoric
9. sensory

Figure 89:  Hemispheric Processes

When a disorder of language results from brain damage, the clinical condition is APHASIA. Aphasia is distinguishable from non-linguistic disorders of speech resulting from weakness or incoordination of the vocal mechanism -- dysarthria, apraxia. The exact nature of the brain's function and aphasia has been debated over the years by two theoretical positions: location and antilocation. The locationists, at one end of a continuum, believe specific behaviors are subserved by specific areas of the brain. Antilocationists, at the opposite end of the spectrum, view mental functions as products of the "whole" brain. There are, of course, theories that lie somewhere between the two extremes. Because, historically, the locationist philosophy was the first modern theory and because it serves as a good foundation for the introductory student to understand the brain's role in speech-language, a basic locationist model has been presented.

How the brain functions depends, in part, on what it is asked to do. If a person is asked to repeat the word "cat", the auditory signal is received at the level of the cerebrum in Area 41, the primary auditory cortex (Heschel's gyrus). The message is then sent to the auditory association cortex, Area 22. This area is the most important auditory area for language and is generally known as Wernicke's Area (some texts may refer to Areas 41, 42, and 22 collectively as Wernicke's Area). Here the individual sounds are given meaning and via a transmission line known as the ARCUATE FASCICULUS, the word form is sent around the posterior margin of the sylvian fissure to Area 44 (Broca's Area). The motor area of Broca formulates the appropriate articultory movements necessary to produce the word and this code is sent to the primary volitional motor cortex. Area 4, in turn, innervates the muscles of speech to orally express -- "cat".

If an individual is asked to read the word "cat", the visual signal is received at the cortical level in Areas 17, 18, 19. From these primary and association regions the message is sent to the ANGULAR GYRUS (39). At this major cortical association area, the visual image calls forth an auditory form of the word from Wernicke's Area. The signal is not actually sent to Wernicke's but rather the angular gyrus is capable of visual-auditory association and becomes a shortcut for the message. Once the corresponding auditory segnal is elicited, it passes on to Broca's Area via the arcuate fasciculus and on to Area 4.

To spell the word "cat" when the auditory stimulus is presented, the process again relies on the angular gyrus where it now calls forth a visual image of "cat" for the auditory signal. Researchers, who support the functional locationism of the brain, note that most individuals, when presented a word visually, will also perceive an auditory form of the word. Similarly, if one is asked to spell a word "silently", the visual image is also manifested.

Based on this "normal" process, any damage to Wernicke's, Broca's, or the transmission lines connecting the two areas would result in difficulty understanding or expressing spoken or written language (Figure

90).    Lesions to Wernicke's Area result in impairment of auditory comprehension.    However, the melody and rate of speech is preserved. While the speech may almost sound normal (fluent), the remarkable feature is that it is devoid of content.    This aphasic individual uses meaningless words, like "thing" as a substitution for the desired word. The basic language characteristics of Wernicke's aphasia is:    fluent conversational speech;    abnormal comprehension of spoken language;    repetition of spoken language;    reading aloud; and writing.

| TYPE OF APHASIA | FLUENCY | REPETITION | COMPREHENSION |
| --- | --- | --- | --- |
| Wernicke's Aphasia | fluent | abnormal | abnormal |
| Broca's Aphasia | nonfluent | abnormal | normal |
| Conduction Aphasia | fluent | abnormal | normal |
| Global Aphasia | nonfluent | abnormal | abnormal |

Figure 90:    Aphasia

Broca's aphasia, on the other hand, is characterized by slow, labored, nonfluent speech.    Small grammatical words and endings of words are omitted, suggesting TELEGRAPHIC speech.    Unlike Wernicke's aphasia, this person has adequate auditory comprehension for understanding most conversation.    The ability to comprehend and realize defective expressive speech often results in frustration and anger by such patients. Characteristic of Broca's aphasia are:    nonfluent conversational speech; normal comprehension;    inability to repeat spoken language;    abnormal reading aloud (silent reading for comphrehension may be normal); and abnormal writing.

When the transmission fibers connecting Wernicke and Broca are defective, the result is CONDUCTION APHASIA.    Speech with this disorder is described as fluent and there is normal auditory comprehension. Repetition of spoken language, however, is abnormal as is reading aloud. Reading silently for comprehension is normal but writing is abnormal.

Over the years, researchers and therapists have identified other clinical syndromes of aphasia. Understanding the model presented here and the consequences of lesions to these areas will prepare the introductory student to pursue this subject in greater detail.

## Apraxia

A condition often associated with aphasia is APRAXIA. Some forms of apraxia described in the literature, for example VERBAL APRAXIA (APRAXIA OF SPEECH), are difficult to differentiate from Broca's aphasia. It is important to remember that apraxia of speech is a speech disturbance, not a disturbance of language. Such patients are capable of producing sounds correctly, but may not be able to do so upon command. Their speech is often characterized by inconsistent articulation with normal comprehension and writing skills. Lesions located on the superior margin of the sylvian fissure (front-parietal operculum) result in BUCCO-FACIAL APRAXIA. This condition is often found with conduction aphasia and Broca's aphasia. It results in the inability of the patient to carry out commands involving the facial and articulatory muscles. Commands such as "stick out your tongue" or "whistle" cannot be fulfilled on a voluntary basis.

## Conclusion

Numerous models have been designed to explain the dynamic processes of the brain and language function. One concept relegated to a philosophical hypothetical construct has been the separation of the brain from the mind and thought. Students are taught that all our functions are dependent on and exclusively tied to events. Mental events are no different than neural motor events. What transpires when we contemplate an action? What are the mental events that cause neural events? The 17th century hypothesis of dualism (mind vs. material world and brain) has again taken on new meaning.

Recent studies with both humans and animals suggest that certain neural activity in the SUPPLEMENTARY MOTOR AREA, which is located on the surface of the cerebral cortex, precedes motor cortex firings by .1 to 1.0 seconds. Some noted physiologists believe this type of research is positively answering the question of whether or not mind and thought exist independently from other neural processes such as those involved in volitional movement. Stated more simply, there may be a master control system, one that is uniquely different from the neuron network resulting in individual performance.

Linguists have drawn a marked distinction between language performance and language competence. Performance is the setting into action; competence comprises the rules that are translated into performance. One can describe language performance, but it is difficult to reconcile the neural processes involved in the theoretical framework of language

competence.    Now,    research  is  on  the  edge  of  relating  language
performance to competence.  Mental events cause neural events.

   The confusion experienced  by many who are students  trying to understand the brain and  its role in governing human behavior  is both frus-
trating  and  exciting.   Research is  making ever increasing  strides in
helping us know ourselves better.  It is hoped that the information presented in  this text to  expand the  students' knowledge of  anatomy and
physiology  will  assist in  meeting  the  challenges presented  in  the
speech-language-hearing profession.

# Glossary

**afferent:**    Refers to nerves which convey sensory impulses from the periphery to the CNS.

**agnosia:**    Loss of the function of recognition of individual sensory stimuli.

**agraphia:**    Inability to express thoughts in writing, due to a lesion in the CNS.

**alogia:**    Inability to speak due to a lesion in the CNS or mental impairment.

**anarthria:**    Inability to articulate due to brain lesion, or to damage to peripheral nerves which innervate the articulatory muscles.

**aphemia:**    Inability to speak due to a lesion in the CNS, or aphasia.

**asymmetrical tonic neck reflex:**    The "fencing position".  Turning the head to the right facilitates the extensor muscles in that side of the body, and increases tone of the flexors of arms and legs in the left side.

**Babinski Reflex:**    Extension of the big toe with fanning of the other toes when the sole is stimulated.

**bulbar:**    Pertaining to the medulla oblongata, the bulb of nervous tissue continuous above with the spinal cord.

**choreoathetosis:**    In CP, slow writing movement of athetosis which is accompanied by a quick component.

**decussation:**    The crossing of nerve tracts in their course to or from lower centers of the brain. (CNS)

**dysphasia:**    Partial or complete loss of the ability to speak or to comprehend the spoken word due to injury, disease, or maldevelopment of the brain.

**efferent:**    Refers to nerves which convey motor impulses from the CNS to the muscles.

**electroencephalograph:**    An instrument for graphically recording electrical currents developed in the cerebral cortex during brain functioning; EEG.

**encephalitis:**    Inflammation of the brain or its membranous envelopes.

**hemiplegia:**    Paralysis of one side of the body.

lesion:    An injury or wound; deficit of tissue.

meningitis:    Inflammation of the three membranes which envelope the brain and spinal cord; the Dura Mater, Pia Mater, and Arachnoid Mater.

Moro Reflex:    The startle reflex; precipitated by sudden noise and characterized by extensor muscle reaction.

neurophrenia:    Behavior symptoms resulting from CNS impairment.

primitive reflex:    Those reflexes normally present at birth, that disappear to allow voluntary movement and posture.

quadriplegia:    Paralysis involving all four extremities.

symmetrical tonic relfex:    In response to flexion of the neck, the flexor muscles of the arms and extensor muscles of the legs are innervated.  When the neck is extended, the extensors of the arms and flexors of the legs are flacilitated.

tonic labryinthine reflex:    The position of the body in space affects muscle tone.  Lying supine (face up), there is an increased tone of all extensor muscles.  Lying prone (face down), there is an increased tone in the flexor muscles.

## References

Baker, P. F. (1975).  The nerve axon.  Scientific American, 212, 74-82.

Chusid, J.G. (1976).  Correlative neuroanatomy and functional neurology (16th ed.).  Los Altos, CA: Lange Medical.

Darley, F. L. (1982).  Aphasia.  Philadelphia: Saunders.

Eccles, J. (1965). The synapse.  Scientific American, 212, 56-66.

Eccles, J. (1982).  Beyond the brain.  Omni, 5, 56-62.  Gardner, E. (1975).  Fundamentals of neurology (6th ed.).  Philadelphia: Saunders.

Goldberg, S. (1979).  Clinical neuroanatomy.  Miami: Med Master.

# INDEX